A Consumer Food Data System for 2030 and Beyond

Panel on Improving Consumer Data for Food and Nutrition Policy Research for the Economic Research Service

Committee on National Statistics

Division of Behavioral and Social Sciences and Education

A Consensus Study Report of

The National Academies of
SCIENCES • ENGINEERING • MEDICINE

THE NATIONAL ACADEMIES PRESS
Washington, DC
www.nap.edu

THE NATIONAL ACADEMIES PRESS 500 Fifth Street, NW Washington, DC 20001

This activity was supported by a contract between the National Academy of Sciences and the Economic Research Service of the U.S. Department of Agriculture under project number 58-5000-7-0106. Support for the work of the Committee on National Statistics is provided by a consortium of federal agencies through a grant from the National Science Foundation, a National Agricultural Statistics Service cooperative agreement, and several individual contracts. Any opinions, findings, conclusions, or recommendations expressed in this publication do not necessarily reflect the views of any organization or agency that provided support for the project.

International Standard Book Number-13: 978-0-309-67071-5
International Standard Book Number-10: 0-309-67071-3
Digital Object Identifier: https://doi.org/10.17226/25657

Additional copies of this publication are available from the National Academies Press, 500 Fifth Street, NW, Keck 360, Washington, DC 20001; (800) 624-6242 or (202) 334-3313; http://www.nap.edu.

Printed in the United States of America

Suggested citation: National Academies of Sciences, Engineering, and Medicine. (2020). *A Consumer Food Data System for 2030 and Beyond*. Washington, DC: The National Academies Press. https://doi.org/10.17226/25657.

The National Academies of

SCIENCES • ENGINEERING • MEDICINE

The **National Academy of Sciences** was established in 1863 by an Act of Congress, signed by President Lincoln, as a private, nongovernmental institution to advise the nation on issues related to science and technology. Members are elected by their peers for outstanding contributions to research. Dr. Marcia McNutt is president.

The **National Academy of Engineering** was established in 1964 under the charter of the National Academy of Sciences to bring the practices of engineering to advising the nation. Members are elected by their peers for extraordinary contributions to engineering. Dr. John L. Anderson is president.

The **National Academy of Medicine** (formerly the Institute of Medicine) was established in 1970 under the charter of the National Academy of Sciences to advise the nation on medical and health issues. Members are elected by their peers for distinguished contributions to medicine and health. Dr. Victor J. Dzau is president.

The three Academies work together as the **National Academies of Sciences, Engineering, and Medicine** to provide independent, objective analysis and advice to the nation and conduct other activities to solve complex problems and inform public policy decisions. The National Academies also encourage education and research, recognize outstanding contributions to knowledge, and increase public understanding in matters of science, engineering, and medicine.

Learn more about the National Academies of Sciences, Engineering, and Medicine at **www.nationalacademies.org.**

PANEL ON IMPROVING CONSUMER DATA FOR FOOD AND NUTRITION POLICY RESEARCH FOR THE ECONOMIC RESEARCH SERVICE

MARIANNE P. BITLER (*Chair*), University of California, Davis
TIM BEATTY, University of California, Davis
SOFIA BERTO VILLAS-BOAS, University of California, Berkeley
F. JAY BREIDT, Colorado State University
CRAIG GUNDERSEN, University of Illinois at Urbana-Champaign
MICHAEL W. LINK, Abt Associates
BRUCE D. MEYER, The University of Chicago
AMY B. O'HARA, Georgetown University
ERIC B. RIMM, Harvard T.H. Chan School of Public Health
NORA CATE SCHAEFFER, University of Wisconsin–Madison
DIANE W. SCHANZENBACH, Northwestern University
PARKE E. WILDE, Tufts University
JAMES P. ZILIAK, University of Kentucky

CHRISTOPHER MACKIE, *Senior Program Officer*
NANCY KIRKENDALL, *Senior Program Officer*
MICHAEL SIRI, *Associate Program Officer*

COMMITTEE ON NATIONAL STATISTICS

Acknowledgments

This Consensus Study Report is the product of contributions from many colleagues whom we thank for their generous time and effort and expert guidance. The project was sponsored by the U.S. Department of Agriculture's (USDA's) Economic Research Service (ERS) to provide guidance to its Food Economics Division as it continues development of key national data sources for measuring the food and nutrition conditions faced by consumers, and the factors that affect those conditions. Work by the Food Economics Division is crucial in helping ERS fulfill its mission to "anticipate trends and emerging issues in agriculture, food, the environment, and rural America and to conduct high-quality, objective economic research to inform and enhance public and private decision making." The efforts of the people listed here enabled the panel to execute its charge to provide guidance to ERS for advancing its Consumer Food Data System (CFDS) over the next 10 years in a way that enhances its capacity to support research and inform current and anticipated policy questions.

The panel thanks ERS staff who attended open meetings and generously gave of their time to present material to inform the panel's deliberations. They provided comprehensive information about the agency's current projects and priorities related to the CFDS. These presentations informed panel members about key developments—exploiting proprietary data, developing linkages across data sources, adding supplements to exiting surveys, and continuing the planning of surveys such as FoodAPS—enabling continued progress on the ERS data infrastructure.

Mary Bohman, administrator (former), Jay Variyam, division director, and Mark Denbaly, deputy division director for Food Economics Data, outlined goals of the study and detailed the agency's blueprint for the current CFDS. Throughout the duration of the study, Jay and Mark provided substantive input and kept the panel up to date on developments at ERS and with FoodAPS and other programs. In documenting the agency's current data programs and research activities, David Levin and Megan Sweitzer, both ERS economists, provided an overview of the use of proprietary data in the CFDS. Andrea Carlson, also an ERS economist, described agency efforts to link nutrition information to other data sources. Shelly Ver Ploeg, chief, Food Assistance Branch, discussed the role of data linking in informing research on how food store access and the larger food environment impact food choices, diet, and diet-related health. Mark Prell, senior economist, presented on the Next Generation Data Platform for using administrative data. Elina Page, ERS economist, provided a detailed overview of FoodAPS and discussed plans for the second round of the survey. Abigail Okrent, ERS research economist, documented current uses of commercial data by ERS and outlined plans for expanding their use. Biing-Hwan Lin, senior economist, presented information on the agency's work linking the Food Availability Data System (FADS) to nutrition intake data from the Agricultural Research Service and National Center for Health Statistics to monitor and research the health and dietary outcomes. ERS research economists Brandon Restrepo and Eliana Zeballos and social science analyst Alisha Coleman-Jensen detailed the use of specialized modules added to federal surveys to advance the CFDS.

The panel also benefited greatly from a number of presentations by experts from beyond the statistical system. Addressing commercial data sources used by USDA, Brian Burke, IRI, described work by his firm with proprietary household and retail scanner price data; Ann Hanson and Louis Lesce, NPD, presented on that company's consumer spending and consumption data collections; and Joseph Fortson of Nielsen described their store-level database of retailers selling consumer packaged goods, including food. The panel also learned a great deal about efforts to combine data sources to advance food and nutrition policy and research. Alison Krester of ILSI North America and Kyle McKillop of the University of Maryland Joint Institute for Food Safety and Nutrition, presented on the USDA Branded Food Products Database, which augments the USDA National Nutrient Database with nutrient composition and ingredient information. Laurie May and Tom Krenzke kept the panel informed about progress on FoodAPS-2, which their company, Westat, is contracted to develop and field. Working with panel member Parke Wilde, Mehreen Ismail of Tufts University summarized strengths and weaknesses of FoodAPS from a researcher perspective and offered suggestions for improvements. Robert Moffitt, Johns Hopkins University, addressed data needs to advance research on program outcomes, food expenditure, reporting errors, and

SNAP impacts, thereby providing insights about productive future directions for ERS surveys. Susan Krebs-Smith, chief, Risk Factor Monitoring and Methods Branch, National Cancer Institute, described the use of USDA consumer food data for health research. Melissa Abelev, assistant deputy administrator at USDA's Food and Nutrition Service described her agency's role in producing and using CFDS information. Several researchers presented ideas for improving food and nutrition data—including integration of commercial and administrative data—for the purpose of informing policy issues. Colleen Heflin, Syracuse University, presented on the insights that can be gleaned by linking SNAP administrative data with other types of administrative data and limitations to this. Justine Hastings, Brown University, discussed her work using retail panel loyalty card data and Rhode Island state administrative records to analyze how SNAP benefits are spent. Charles Courtemanche, University of Kentucky, presented work assessing the quality of administrative SNAP data used in FoodAPS. Rachel Shattuck, chief, Survey Improvement Research Branch of the Census Bureau, presented on the quality and utility of an interagency cooperative program called the Next-Generation Data Platform. John Eltinge, assistant director at the U.S. Census Bureau, presented information to the panel about interagency efforts to address quality issues associated with using multiple data sources (including proprietary data). Cordell Golden, statistician at the National Center for Health Statistics, described ongoing record linkage programs at his agency. Rob Santos, vice president and chief methodologist, The Urban Institute, described nongovernment sources for filling data gaps in the CFDS, including those produced through a collaboration with the Feeding America program. Alessandro Bonanno, Colorado State University, presented ideas for improving geospatial information in ERS's food data system. On the topic of using proprietary data for food policy research, Mary Muth, director of RTI's Food, Nutrition, and Obesity Policy Research Program, described types, sources, and considerations and limitations in using store scanner data, household scanner data, and nutrition data from labels for food policy research. On a related topic, Helen Jensen, Iowa State, described how proprietary scanner data could help shed light on issues related to the WIC program. Carma Hogue, assistant division chief, U.S. Census Bureau, described that agency's work on improving economic statistics through web scraping and machine learning. Finally, the panel heard presentations informing the panel about data needs for implementation and assessment of programs at state and local levels. Shannon Whaley, director, Research and Evaluation, PHFE WIC (Public Health Foundation Enterprises, Special Supplemental Nutrition Program for Women Infants and Children)—the largest local WIC agency in the country—discussed data needs for planning, development, and evaluation of programs designed to promote the healthy development of low-income children and families.

Caroline Danielson, policy director and senior fellow, Public Policy Institute of California, presented data needs for effective administration of state-level programs such as SNAP/Calfresh. Wendi Gosliner, unit director, Nutrition Policy Institute, University of California, discussed data needs for research and policy to improve federal food and nutrition programs, such as WIC and SNAP-Ed, designed to improve population health. Hilary Hoynes, professor, Public Policy and Economics, University of California, Berkeley, discussed the role of different kinds of data, including administrative data and data on policy choices made by states, for understanding health outcomes associated with programs such as SNAP and WIC.

The panel could not have conducted its work efficiently without the capable staff of the National Academies of Sciences, Engineering, and Medicine: Brian Harris-Kojetin, director, Committee on National Statistics, provided institutional leadership and substantive contributions during meetings. Kirsten Sampson-Snyder, director of reports, Division of Behavioral and Social Sciences and Education, expertly coordinated the review process; and Marc DeFrancis provided thorough final editing that improved the readability of the report for a wide audience. We also thank Michael Siri, senior program associate, for his well-organized and efficient logistical support of the panel's meetings, as well as his contribution to assembling and formatting of this report. Nancy Kirkendall was essential in drafting important sections of the report and providing insights based on her long experience with USDA data and research issues and with the U.S. statistical system. On behalf of the panel, I thank the study director, Christopher Mackie, for his tireless work and enthusiasm, which propelled us forward.

Finally, and most importantly, a note of appreciation is in order for my fellow panel members. This report reflects the collective expertise and commitment of all panel members: Tim Beatty, Department of Agricultural and Resource Economics, University of California, Davis; Sofia Berto Villas-Boas, Department of Agricultural and Resource Economics, University of California, Berkeley; F. Jay Breidt, Department of Statistics, Colorado State University; Craig Gundersen, Department of Agricultural and Consumer Economics, University of Illinois; Michael Link, Division for Data Science, Surveys & Enabling Technologies, Abt Associates; Bruce D. Meyer, Harris School of Public Policy Studies, The University of Chicago; Amy O'Hara, McCourt School of Public Policy, Georgetown University; Eric B. Rimm, Department of Epidemiology and Department of Nutrition, Harvard T.H. Chan School of Public Health; Nora Cate Schaeffer, Department of Sociology, University of Wisconsin–Madison; Diane W. Schanzenbach, Institute for Policy Research and School of Education and Social Policy, Northwestern University; Parke E. Wilde, Friedman School of Nutrition Science and Policy, Tufts University; and James P. Ziliak, Center for Poverty Research, University of Kentucky. This group—chosen for their diverse perspectives, backgrounds, and subject matter knowledge—gave generously of their time to attend meetings and to apply their expertise in the writing of this report.

This Consensus Study Report was reviewed in draft form by individuals chosen for their diverse perspectives and technical expertise. The purpose of this independent review is to provide candid and critical comments that will assist the National Academies in making each published report as sound as possible and to ensure that it meets the institutional standards for quality, objectivity, evidence, and responsiveness to the study charge. The review comments and draft manuscript remain confidential to protect the integrity of the deliberative process.

We thank the following individuals for their review of this report: Scott W. Allard, Evans School of Public Policy and Governance, University of Washington; Alessandro Bonanno, Department of Agricultural and Resource Economics, Colorado State University; Alicia L. Carriquiry, Department of Statistics, Iowa State University; Randy Green, Food and Agriculture and Public Affairs, Watson Green, LLC, Washington, DC; Danny O. Jacobs, President's Office, Oregon Health Sciences University; Barbara A. Laraia, School of Public Health, University of California, Berkeley; William Layden, School of Public Health, Indiana University; Robert A. Moffitt, Department of Economics, Johns Hopkins University; Mary K. Muth, Food and Agricultural Policy Research, RTI International; and Robert L. Santos, Chief Methodologist's Office, The Urban Institute.

Although the reviewers listed above provided many constructive comments and suggestions, they were not asked to endorse the conclusions or recommendations, nor did they see the final draft of the report before its release. The review of the report was overseen by Mary Ellen Bock (professor emeritus), Purdue University, and Barbara Schaal, professor, Washington University in St. Louis. They were responsible for making certain that an independent examination of this report was carried out in accordance with the standards of the National Academies and that all review comments were carefully considered. Responsibility for the final content rests entirely with the authoring committee and the National Academies.

Marianne P. Bitler, *Chair*
Panel on Improving Consumer Data for Food and Nutrition Policy Research for the Economic Research Service

Contents

Summary

The Food Economics Division of the U.S. Department of Agriculture's (USDA's) Economic Research Service (ERS) engages in research and data collection to inform policy making related to the leading federal nutrition assistance programs managed by USDA's Food and Nutrition Service (FNS).[1] ERS also studies how food consumption and nutrition influence the U.S. population's health and well-being, which in turn affect the cost of government health insurance programs. Food insecurity and inadequate nutrition are strongly associated with a range of health and social consequences, including acute birth outcomes, impaired academic performance, and behavioral control and acuity problems. Understanding why people choose foods, how food assistance programs affect these choices, and what the health impacts are must be informed by a multisource, interconnected, reliable data system. In conducting these data collection and research activities, ERS advances the public good.

The Consumer Food Data System (CFDS) is a "portfolio of data resources that measure, from the perspective of a consumer, food and nutrition conditions. and the factors that affect those conditions" (Larimore et al., 2018). It supports stand-alone surveys and specialized modules

[1]As stated by the agency, "FED [food economics division] conducts economic research and analysis on policy-relevant issues related to the food sector (food safety, food prices, and markets); consumer behavior related to food choices (food consumption, diet quality, and nutrition); and food and nutrition assistance programs (SNAP, WIC, National School Lunch Program). FED also provides data and statistics on food prices, food expenditures, and the food supply chain." See https://www.ers.usda.gov/about-ers/agency-structure/food-economics-division-fed.

added to established federal surveys, and it links USDA-funded survey data to external sources, including other survey data; commercial data; and federal, state, and local government administrative data. The CFDS helps the agency fulfill its mission to "anticipate trends and emerging issues in agriculture, food, the environment, and rural America and to conduct high-quality, objective economic research to inform and enhance public and private decision making."[2]

ERS asked the National Academies of Sciences, Engineering, and Medicine's Committee on National Statistics to review and provide guidance for its CFDS program. The key component of the charge (reproduced in full in Chapter 1) was to provide a blueprint for increasing the value of the CFDS by "providing guidance for its advancement over the next 10 years" to enhance its capacity to support research that informs high-priority current and future policy questions. The charge also asked for guidance regarding future iterations of ERS's National Household Food Acquisition and Purchase Survey (FoodAPS), which was the first comprehensive survey on food acquisitions from all sources.

THE SCOPE OF A CONSUMER FOOD AND NUTRITION DATA SYSTEM

High-quality, comprehensive data (i) produce *descriptive information* about population and program characteristics, (ii) serve a *monitoring function* to track nutrition, health, food security and safety, and other outcomes, and (iii) support research, including *causal inference and program evaluation*.

Descriptive information about food and nutrition safety net programs and the healthfulness of U.S. diets is important in its own right. Monitoring information provides a series of snapshots of outcomes nationally and, when available, at more granular state and local levels. Examples of questions answered through careful data monitoring include: How many people have limited access to sources of healthy and affordable foods? What is the healthfulness of the American diet? Who participates in USDA food assistance programs? How do food security and obesity change over time? And, in what ways are Supplemental Nutrition Assistance Program (SNAP) and low-income households similar to or different from the overall population?

The third functional role of the CFDS is to enable USDA staff and outside researchers to answer causal questions about important food-related outcomes. For example, how does access to grocery stores, restaurants, and the broader food environment affect food choices and diet-related health?

[2] See https://www.ers.usda.gov/about-ers.

And, how do SNAP, the Special Supplemental Nutrition Program for Women, Infant, and Children (WIC), and school meals programs and policies affect nutrition, food security, health, and use of health care systems?

Features of a (nonexperimental) data system that facilitate strong causal research designs include (i) the provision of sampling frames through administrative data that can be used for random assignment or survey purposes; (ii) the provision of comparison data that are nationally representative for use in understanding the study populations through nonexperimental evaluations; (iii) integration with policy information as explanatory variables (as is emphasized in parts of this report that address the SNAP rules); (iv) longitudinal or panel structures for use in fixed-effects models that control for unobserved time-constant confounding variables; and (v) inclusion of appropriate administrative data on program participation linked with nationally or regionally representative survey or administrative data on the population of potentially eligible persons.

DESIRABLE CHARACTERISTICS OF A CONSUMER FOOD AND NUTRITION DATA SYSTEM

Recognizing that tradeoffs must be made, the panel identified several characteristics of a data system that are desirable in terms of its usefulness for research and informing policy:

- **Comprehensiveness.** To monitor levels and trends in food behaviors and related outcomes and to identify the effects of public programs and policies on those behaviors, a comprehensive data system requires a variety of sources spanning multiple topics.
- **Representativeness.** Data on food behaviors and outcomes are most useful if it is representative of the U.S. population, both nationally and subnationally.
- **Timeliness.** To have maximum program and policy impact, the system collects data at regular intervals, repeats over time at an appropriate frequency, and releases data without undue delay.
- **Openness.** Because data programs are maintained with taxpayer funds, data should be accessible to the public and to the research community. Security and privacy concerns must be addressed before making de-identified data available.
- **Flexibility.** A flexible data system recognizes that food and consumer data will be used for some research applications that were planned in advance, as well as for applications generated by a broad, entrepreneurial, and inventive community of research users studying unanticipated changes in policy, food retail markets, or consumer preferences.

- **Accuracy.** Accurate measurement and reporting are the foundation of effective evidence-based policy making, so a desirable data system is one that seeks continuous quality improvement. Given increased reliance on data produced by state and local governments and commercial entities for purposes other than scientific study, continual assessment and improvement of the quality of these sources will be a central part of the CFDS.
- **Suitability for causal analysis.** While some policy questions can be answered with descriptive information, others require cause-and-effect inference. With this in mind, data design efforts should include (i) the collection and sharing of policy variables for use in implementing quasi-experimental designs, (ii) the use of administrative data for potential program evaluations with random-assignment research designs, and (iii) the creation of longitudinal survey and administrative data (either repeated cross-sections or panel data) for use in statistical analyses that offer causal insight.
- **Fiscal responsibility.** The CFDS should maximize the research value of federal dollars invested in the data system (including staff time) through its combined impact in descriptive information, monitoring functions, and estimation of causal effects.

Achieving these characteristics in a data system to support food and nutrition research requires a multipronged approach involving survey, administrative, and commercial data (Larimore et al., 2018).

EXPLOITING DIVERSE SOURCES OF DATA

The federal government's statistical system—a survey-centric one reflecting best methodological practices of the 20th century—is now at a crossroads. Declining response rates have led to surveys becoming ever more costly and, at times, less accurate and generalizable. This well-documented development (Commission on Evidence-Based Policymaking, 2017; NASEM, 2017a), coupled with the emergence of lower-burden complementary and alternative data sources, has given rise to new data paradigms. The CFDS is well positioned in this changing data environment given its advances in blending surveys, administrative data (residing within USDA programs or elsewhere, such as the Census Bureau), and proprietary commercial data (including retail scanner data, household scanner data, and geospatial information on food stores and restaurants).

Although recent changes in the kinds of data available for research purposes have been profound, surveys continue to play an essential role. Some information, such as nutrition outcomes, cannot be acquired from administrative or other nonsurvey data sources. Traditionally, surveys have also been the main source for data on eligibility, participation, and benefit amounts for safety net programs such as SNAP, WIC, and Temporary Assistance for Needy Families; but there are concerns about respondent burden and data accuracy for these purposes (Meyer et al., 2015). Administrative data residing within government agencies, sometimes linked to survey data, can provide accurate measures of program participation and benefit amounts. Commercial data—obtained directly from food vendors or from companies engaged as third-party private aggregators, such as Nielsen and IRI—have become increasingly desirable because of the high volume, detail, and frequency of information they can provide about food prices, food outlets, and the spectrum of food choices within those outlets. However, by their nature, commercial data are not designed for research purposes, and they are typically only made available under restrictive arrangements. Nonetheless,

> **RECOMMENDATION 4.2: To make effective use of limited resources for survey investments, the U.S. Department of Agriculture should further exploit both administrative data sources and commercial data sources for applications in which they can be effectively used.**

The high value to USDA's CFDS created by linkages to external datasets—whether commercial or administrative—is enhanced when data cover parallel concepts in the same geographic areas across time, allowing for an evaluation of the effects of policy changes and other interventions.

IMPROVING SURVEY COMPONENTS OF THE CFDS

As described in Chapter 2, USDA invests in multiple survey data sources, including (i) modules on major nationally representative surveys fielded by other government agencies, (ii) survey components in FNS-supported evaluation studies, and (iii) the partnership between ERS and FNS to create FoodAPS. FoodAPS provides descriptive data on where households acquire food in a typical week, which foods they acquire, and how much they pay (Todd and Scharadin, 2016). It is unique among data sources in tracking both food acquired to eat at home and food acquired away from home. It allows analyses that examine which factors are correlated with households' decisions about where to shop for food (Ver Ploeg et al., 2017); which household characteristics are associated with increased childhood obesity risks (Jo, 2017); how SNAP benefits are used over the course of the benefit month (Smith et al., 2016); and how price variation across geographic areas is associated with food choices and whether this varies by SNAP participation (Basu et al., 2016). FoodAPS supports monitoring functions by allowing the choices of program recipients and eligible nonrecipients of food assistance programs to be examined. Although the cross-sectional design imposes limitations, FoodAPS has also spawned some causal impact research. For example, Kuhn (2018) examines the impact of Electronic Benefit Transfers (EBT) on households' intramonth consumption cycles.

A key innovation of FoodAPS is its use of linkages to nonsurvey data sources. One example of this design element is the use of official SNAP administrative records to create a frame for sampling SNAP recipients. Information on nutrient intake and the retail environment was added using commercially produced barcodes, product descriptions, and household location data.

The development and fielding of FoodAPS encountered the usual high level of technical burden associated with creating a new dataset with many linkages. Since FoodAPS cannot satisfy all analytic demands, resource allocation for it needs to be assigned in a way that leaves resources available for other data programs. Because the greatest strength of FoodAPS is in its capacity to generate descriptive and monitoring information for research and policy, and also because it is an expensive survey, it is not practical to envision it as an annual or even biannual program. That said, there is clear value to conducting the survey on a regular basis, because doing so would allow it to contribute to the construction of stylized facts for the monitoring function of the CFDS. Implementing a fixed and predictable schedule (e.g., as the Census Bureau does with the Economic Census) would generate efficiencies and predictability by creating a regular staffing cycle for the Food and Economics Division (FED). This is important if ERS is to manage the data system without having other valuable components of the CFDS suffer when FoodAPS's resource demands are high.

RECOMMENDATION 4.3: The National Household Food Acquisition and Purchase Survey (FoodAPS) should be conducted on a regular schedule, such as once every 5 years.

The move to a regular schedule would also allow ERS to plan for the integration of new data sources, such as administrative data on multiple programs. The ordered planning cycle would facilitate continual process improvement and strengthen institutional memory of how a national survey is conducted. This approach would also avoid the need to pay the fixed costs of conducting new surveys at uneven time intervals. Finally, asking consistent questions over time would also improve the usefulness of the resulting data by, for example, allowing for comparability across assessments of time trends.

To the extent that FoodAPS is intended to support research beyond the monitoring of food acquisitions and related outcomes, such as longitudinal and causal research, planners can learn from other surveys that match samples to longitudinal administrative data. While, for cost and other reasons, a true longitudinal structure is not feasible for FoodAPS, the survey could sample from the same geographical units—that is, the same primary sampling units (PSUs)—to create a repeated cross-sectional design. This would permit researchers to combine cross-PSU changes over time in socioeconomic conditions, policy choices, and the built environment to assess how economic, policy, and environmental factors affect food acquisition and related outcomes collected in FoodAPS.

RECOMMENDATION 4.4: The National Household Food Acquisition and Purchase Survey (FoodAPS) should be reviewed across a set of design dimensions for future iterations. Along with linkages to extant administrative records from other federal and state statistical agencies, the review should assess the efficacy of sampling from the same set of primary sampling units over time to facilitate more rigorous monitoring and evaluation functions.

More broadly within the survey domain, ERS has made effective use of modules attached to other surveys. Examples include the Food Security Supplement (in the Current Population Survey), the Flexible Consumer Behavior Survey (in the National Health and Nutrition Examination Survey[3] [NHANES]), and the Eating and Health Module (in the American Time Use Survey). This approach, which ERS will no doubt continue to pursue, allows the strengths of established instruments, such as the set of explanatory covariates contained therein, to be exploited.

USE OF ADMINISTRATIVE DATA IN THE CFDS

Statistical agencies are investing more heavily in administrative data sources than they have in the past, for reasons to do with both the high cost of survey approaches and the accuracy of information. Administrative data can be used in a variety of ways, both on their own and in combination with other data. The case for expanded and better coordinated use of valuable administrative data—such as those that reside within federal, state, and local governments—is especially clear for purposes of program monitoring, evaluation, and improvement. This value is enhanced when the administrative records can be linked to data

[3]NHANES is the only food intake survey in the United States. Because it is designed to collect information on consumers' "knowledge, attitudes, and beliefs regarding nutrition and food choices," it relates to many of the issues that fall within FED's purview. See https://www.ers.usda.gov/topics/food-choices-health/food-consumption-demand/flexible-consumer-behavior-survey.

on the population of program eligibles, such as from sources such as the American Community Survey.

ERS has improved its capacity to collaborate across agencies, in part through a Census Bureau and USDA partnership—the Next Generation Data Platform—that allows the agency to access and analyze detailed SNAP participation data from many states and WIC data from several states. Subsequent linkages to survey data have improved USDA models of SNAP eligibility and participation rates (Scherpf et al., 2015). Using the Next Generation tools, the linked survey and program records have been found to more accurately reflect information about participants than the survey data alone. For this program, ERS relies on the Census Bureau's infrastructure to negotiate sharing arrangements and to ingest, harmonize, and link records.

Another area with great potential for enhancing research is the expansion of access to policy databases maintained by several nutrition programs. For example, the SNAP Policy Database includes information on a host of SNAP policy choices, and the SNAP Distribution Database contains information on the timing of SNAP distributions by different states within the month. These are models of administrative data resources that allow research to be carried out on policy options, such as how different choices made by different governmental entities affect outcomes in their localities. These databases also enable research on the causal effects of program participation using the SNAP cycle.

RECOMMENDATION 4.13: The Supplemental Nutrition Assistance Program (SNAP) Policy Database and the SNAP Distribution Database should be updated annually by the Economic Research Service's (ERS's) Food and Economics Division. Similar cross-state over-time policy databases on additional food assistance programs, such as Special Supplemental Nutrition Program for Women, Infants, and Children (WIC), the School Breakfast Program, the National School Lunch Program, and the Child and Adult Care Food Program should be established and updated annually by ERS. Data that measure rules affecting participating retailers (e.g., stocking requirements) and other entities (e.g., reimbursed foods in school meals programs) should also be collected and made available. Data should be made available about the geographic location of benefit offices (e.g., the city, county, state, latitude, and longitude of locations where participants apply and recertify for assistance, including schools, SNAP offices, and WIC clinics). Finally, administrative data on store participation in SNAP (through the Store Tracking and Redemption System) and WIC (through The Integrity Profile) should be made available with geographic locations

for participating retailers; the possibility of making redemption data available should also be explored.

Ideally, data would be included on cash purchases and SNAP or WIC redemptions for the same individuals and sales and redemptions at the same stores so complete acquisitions could be studied.

Recent legislative developments provide support for ERS as it moves to maximize the potential of administrative data. The Foundations for Evidence-Based Policymaking Act states, "the head of an agency shall, to the extent practicable, make any data asset maintained by the agency available, upon request, to any statistical agency or unit for purposes of developing evidence." And the Farm Bill states that the Secretary shall provide guidance and direction on how states should form longitudinal databases supporting research on participation in and the operation of SNAP.

RECOMMENDATION 4.7: To aid the Economic Research Service (ERS) in expanding the Next Generation Data platform, intergovernmental coordination is needed to maximize the impacts of infrastructure changes made by the Farm Bill (the Agricultural Improvement Act of 2018) and the Foundations for Evidence-Based Policymaking Act. States and localities should share their administrative data, including the Supplemental Nutrition Assistance Program and Special Supplemental Nutrition Program for Women, Infants, and Children case records, with the U.S. Department of Agriculture (USDA). USDA should optimize use and access through data intermediaries, including but not limited to the Census Bureau. ERS should develop specifications for their process whereby researchers access administrative and commercial data, and for how researcher-provided data can be brought in and linked to other data.

Coordinated data sharing would involve careful assessment of the quality and comparability, across locations, of the administrative data brought in. States and localities have different data systems and records, all of which need to be checked for consistency and harmonized.

ERS's vision for the CFDS should include partnerships within the federal statistical system so that survey data may be blended with administrative or proprietary data with little error. If the Evidence Act makes information from other agencies available to ERS for statistical purposes, administrative data on workforce, housing, justice, and education could be incorporated into ERS studies of program participation. The Evidence Act requires that the Office of Management and Budget (OMB) establish a single application process for access to confidential federal data. Section 3564(f) notes that nothing in that Act preempts applicable state law regarding the confidentiality of data collected by the states. It is expected that OMB and the statistical agencies will gather, interpret, and deconflict any laws and regulations related to data access.

USE OF COMMERCIAL DATA IN THE CFDS

The FED has a strong track record of using proprietary scanner and sales data to estimate detailed food prices and quantities of purchases, retail sales, consumption, and purchases of food for at-home and away-from-home eating. For example, data on consumer purchase transactions and retail point-of-sales and information from food labels have been used to help answer questions about the cost of a healthy diet and about how the nutrient content of food products changes over time.

To fully analyze program participation through changing social, economic, and policy conditions, the use of administrative data alone from those programs is insufficient. Data from surveys and commercial sources can provide more comprehensive information, whether on the full population of households or retailers, to model take-up rates; or to model the population effects of participation on health outcomes; or to model population subgroups, such as veterans. Data available through commercial research organizations or partnerships with commercial food providers are especially useful for improving information about the food environment. Such data can help address critical questions in areas such as (i) dietary patterns and nutrition; (ii) the food environment, including the availability of stores and restaurants, food prices in an area, and community characteristics; and (iii) industry response and agricultural sector adaptations to these many changes (Larimore et al., 2018).

In summary, because of their potential value to research, ERS should continue to invest in acquiring and understanding commercial data.

RECOMMENDATION 4.8: The U.S. Department of Agriculture (USDA) should exploit new ideas for integrating commercial data into the Consumer Food Data System. For example, to produce a long "time series" of data on Supplemental Nutrition Assistance Program (SNAP) participation, food insecurity status, and the location of all stores in the immediate environment of the respondent, USDA could facilitate matching restricted-access Food Security Supplement data (with respondents' locations) with TDLinx data on stores, state data on SNAP and other program participation, and Store Tracking and Redemption System data on stores that redeem SNAP.

As these new sources of data become available for use by food researchers and evaluators, there is also a need for a deep understanding of their strengths and weaknesses. As a general class of data, "organic data," which arise out of the broader information ecosystem, are not designed for research purposes, but can still have great value in part because they tend be massive, with millions or more of observations. They are also often generated in close to "real time" (retail scanner data capture the exact time and date of each scanned transaction), and in a way that is unobtrusive for measuring phenomena since there is no direct engagement with subjects. For example, retail scanner data are captured as part of the natural store checkout process.

While commercial data will certainly play a growing role in food research, measurement, and assessment, hurdles need to be overcome before their full potential can be realized. Chief among these are access, coverage, and transparency issues. Often, one of the most difficult aspects of using commercial data is negotiating access (NASEM, 2017a). For example, while non-ERS-affiliated users can obtain access to retail data from Nielsen through the Kilts Center for Marketing at the University of Chicago's Booth School of Business, they face limitations—for example, to information on precise geographic locations—that impede some kinds of analyses.

Regarding coverage and representation, to obtain valid and reliable conclusions it is critical that the data be representative of the populations or subpopulations of interest and that the degree of representativeness be known. For example, in some commercial databases, lower-income consumers are underrepresented; at the retail level, smaller, independent stores or private-label products may be excluded. In some cases, design data can be used to correct for coverage issues and selection biases in organic data. Additionally, in terms of transparency, organic data often lack the traditional types of documentation researchers are accustomed to having. This applies not only to the data content but also to the ability to trace the origins of the data or changes made to the data at various points before reaching the researcher. For example, the consumer panel widely used by researchers does not collect individual prices paid by consumers when they shop at stores where firm-side data are available; instead, what is reported in the data is the average weekly price from these other sources, sometimes averaged across various geographies.

Overcoming the above hurdles will guide ERS's quest for accurate and applicable data sources.

RECOMMENDATION 4.9: As with survey and administrative data, commercial data in the Consumer Food Data System should be continually reviewed for accuracy. Data checking, including comparing proprietary commercial data with other sources, such as the Census of Retail Trade, is an essential part of data acquisition, data processing, and vetting. It is important to document coverage of these auxiliary

data in terms of geography, the distribution of retail outlets across types, and the amount of purchases captured. It is also important to construct weights to make the population of participants demographically representative of the national population.[4]

For example, ERS has an admirable tradition of using Nielsen and IRI data while also comparing findings, totals, and coverage with other sources and while documenting the strengths and weaknesses of these scanner and sales datasets. Often, ERS-funded work is the sole source of information about the accuracy of these proprietary data.

DATA QUALITY AND DATA ACCESS

ERS must continue to envision a future when there is much more blending of mixed data types. Whenever a major survey such as FoodAPS is designed, the role of administrative data or other data types should be considered in the overall design and estimation strategy, and the considerations should include the coverage, quality, timeliness, accessibility, and cost of those data. Even with the inevitable trend toward mixed-data models, surveys will continue to be important to statistical agencies for the foreseeable future. Surveys provide household- and individual-level data that cannot always be acquired through other means.

RECOMMENDATION 4.1: A key task for the Consumer Food Data System is to assess the quality of survey data across sources and over time. This should be done by linking the surveys to auxiliary sources in order to check sample records. For example, work comparing population totals and individual reports of program participation can be done by comparing survey totals to administrative totals and comparing self-reports to administrative records. The level of misreporting in the data and the characteristics of those misreporting should be catalogued.

In the new data paradigm, administrative and commercial data must be evaluated for quality as would-be survey data. As ERS continues to enhance data products through more expansive use of proprietary data and links to state, local, and other federal administrative data, quality assessment will be critical. Other questions that are important for evaluating these sources include: (i) Are the data longitudinal? (ii) Can the changing

[4] Some sources, such as the IRI Consumer Panel, include weights that are provided to ERS as part of the data purchase. Other sources, such as InfoScan data, do not come with weights.

platforms among proprietary providers and state/local program administrators be harmonized? and (iii) Are the internal algorithms used to compile the data transparent?

While standards are emerging for gauging the quality of stand-alone data and of linkages in sources such as those contained in the CFDS, the quality of data can only be thoroughly assessed through their regular use by researchers.

RECOMMENDATION 4.4: The Economic Research Service's (ERS's) Food Economics Division should create a process for hosting restricted-use data through a secure platform such as the Federal Statistical Research Data Centers network. Data for publicly funded programs should be made available for research at granular levels, including individual-level de-identified and linkable data, while still addressing privacy concerns. This should include information generated in activities funded or sponsored by ERS and Food and Nutrition Service, including the food assistance programs and other programs whose output is included in the Consumer Food Data System.

Taking advantage of multiple data sources requires that the ERS FED partner with other agencies to leverage strengths. For example, ERS may decide it is cost-effective to leverage Census survey methodology expertise for some data projects. In other cases, the agency should take advantage of interagency work on developing standards to assess survey and administrative and proprietary data.

RECOMMENDATION 4.15: The Economic Research Service's (ERS's) Food Economics Division should create a data council to prioritize which data should be created and specify access rules while ensuring that the Consumer Food Data System addresses ongoing U.S. Department of Agriculture research data needs. This council should also help create and update a longer-term data-infrastructure plan. This plan should balance two goals. Access should be as wide as possible to facilitate policy making, scientific advances, education and training, and public understanding about society. Yet, at the same time, data stewards are ethically and legally obligated to protect privacy and sensitive attributes. ERS should seek input from the American Statistical Association, the federal statistical system, and the broader data and research community on how to prevent re-identification, protect sensitive attributes, and increase access. This data council could also be tasked with setting and reviewing the rules for access to ERS and/or Federal Statistical Research Data Centers, described above. This approach could follow the model of the Department of Health

and Human Services' data council, and it should include nongovernment stakeholders.

This report presents a series of recommendations that span the current and past CFDS and also makes suggestions for the future. The most important recommendations, not listed in priority order, relate to (i) checking data and linkage quality, (ii) enhancing access to existing data and future data sources by outside researchers as well as through existing relationships, with greater geographic detail, (iii) finding ways to incorporate more administrative data into the CFDS, (iv) systematically focusing on the CFDS role in serving monitoring needs (e.g., measuring food security consistently) and causal research needs through longitudinal designs, and (v) creating policy databases to enhance causal research.

1

Introduction

1.1. WHY MEASURE THE POPULATION'S FOOD INTAKE AND NUTRITION?

Patterns of food consumption and nutritional intake strongly affect the population's health and well-being in the United States, as in every other country. The Economic Research Service (ERS), in part through its Consumer Food Data System (CFDS), advances our understanding of these impacts.[1] Food and nutrition intake influence diverse outcomes, including risk of chronic disease, risk of death, and economic costs. The economic burden of diet-related diseases amounts to trillions of dollars annually: negative outcomes associated with obesity and overweight alone are estimated to cost $1.42 trillion every year ($428 billion in direct expenditures and $989 billion in lost productivity); cardiovascular diseases cost $316 billion ($190 billion in direct expenditures and $126 billion in lost productivity); and type 2 diabetes costs $320 billion ($112 billion in direct expenditures

[1]The agency's mission is "to anticipate trends and emerging issues in agriculture, food, the environment, and rural America and to conduct high-quality, objective economic research to inform and enhance public and private decision making. ERS shapes its research program and products to serve those who routinely make or influence public policy and program decisions. Key clientele include White House and U.S. Department of Agriculture (USDA) policy officials; the U.S. Congress; program administrators and managers; other federal agencies; state and local government officials; and organizations, including farm and industry groups and those studying food assistance. ERS research provides context for and informs the decisions that affect the agricultural sector, which in turn benefits everyone with efficient stewardship of our agricultural resources and the economic prosperity of the sector." See https://www.ers.usda.gov/about-ers.

and $208 billion in lost productivity) (Milken Institute, 2016; Benjamin et al., 2017; Centers for Medicare & Medicaid Services, 2017). Consequently, understanding why people choose foods and how food assistance programs affect these choices is crucial.

ERS research influences real-world policy making and public spending for health insurance and food and nutrition assistance programs, which account for roughly $100 billion in federal spending (Oliveira, 2017). U.S. Department of Agriculture's (USDA's) expenditures on the Supplemental Nutrition Assistance Program (SNAP), formerly the Food Stamps Program, were $70.8 billion in 2016. During a typical month, 42.2 million people participated in SNAP. In the same year, expenditures for the Special Supplemental Nutrition Program for Women, Infants, and Children (WIC) were about $6 billion, and the program served an average of 7.3 million people per month, including some of the country's most vulnerable populations. The program is restricted to pregnant, postpartum, and breastfeeding women and children under age 5. Expenditures on the National School Lunch Program were $14 billion (for an average daily participation of 30 million people), and expenditures on the National School Breakfast Program were $4 billion (for an average daily participation of 15 million people).

Another perspective is offered by thinking about how many people are participating in these programs across their life cycle and not simply at a given point in time. From this perspective, the school meals programs and WIC have very large footprints, with all hot meals at schools being subsidized by the school meals programs and with WIC serving more than half of all infants. With this level of spending and impacts on this many people at stake, it is essential that the design of outcomes-driven policies be as well informed as possible. Investments in the data used to inform those policy choices can yield large returns in program effectiveness.

In an array of health-related policy areas, ERS research on agriculture, food, food assistance programs and the food environment, and nutrition programs advances the public good.

1.2. GOALS OF A CONSUMER FOOD DATA SYSTEM

ERS's vision for its Food Economics Division (FED) is to build a comprehensive, integrated data system to efficiently deliver credible evidence for informing research and policy. Data collection and sampling designs should always be motivated by the important research and policy questions to be answered and take into account possible variations in policy that may affect outcomes either by design or by accident and the characteristics of the targeted and ultimately affected populations. For example, if it is anticipated that research will employ instrumental variables (or other econometric methods for causal inference), then data collection for potential instruments should be considered part of the research task. If it is anticipated that natural experiments based on existing policy variations will be employed, then data on those policy variations become essential.

Along the spectrum of data uses, the CFDS is designed for "monitoring, identifying, and understanding changes in food supply, purchases, and consumption patterns" for individuals, households, and markets (Larimore et al., 2018). Components of the CFDS include population surveys, either stand-alone or as modules added to extant surveys, many of which are fielded by other statistical agencies. They also include administrative data residing within USDA programs and proprietary commercial data, as well as products created by blending across all these sources. The desirable characteristics and qualities of a CFDS, and recommendations for achieving them, are examined in detail in Chapter 4.

The CFDS is structured to track sequential elements of the food supply system, focusing on consumer acquisition. In the food supply system, food (commodities) moves from the agricultural sector (farmers) through food processors and distributors to grocery stores and restaurants (retailers) to reach the ultimate consumer (see Figure 1.1). In return, money flows from the consumer through retailers, processors, and distributors, eventually to reach the ultimate producer. Food assistance programs can alter the relationship between consumers and retailers in a variety of ways, for example depending on whether they offer vouchers for food or directly provide it. Changes

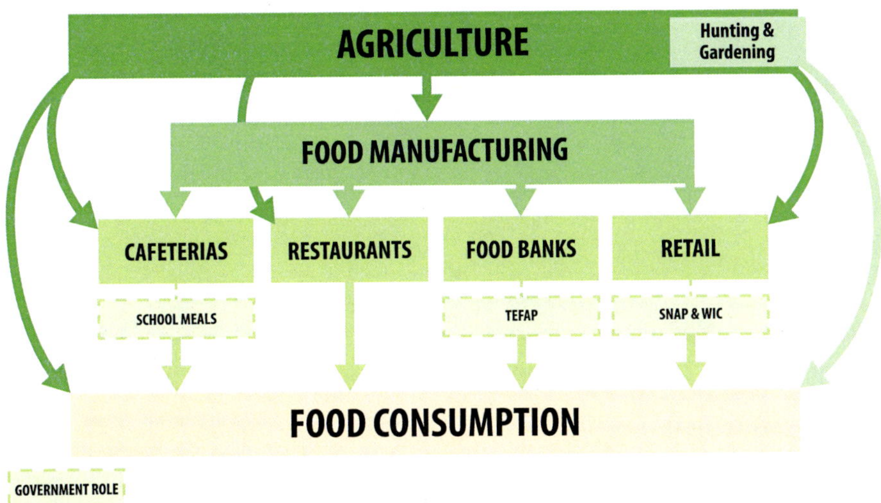

FIGURE 1.1. Food supply system (chain).
NOTES: TEFAP = The Emergency Food Assistance Program.

in supply are reflected through the chain to consumers, and changes in consumption are reflected back through the supply chain to producers. Food losses occur at each transition. Food acquisition obviously affects food consumption, which is the direct link to health and well-being. Thus, understanding the food supply system is a critical part of understanding the health of the economy as well as the health and well-being of the people.

Both the supply and the prices associated with food commodities (e.g., as produced by farmers, represented in Figure 1.1) are measured by the USDA's National Agricultural Statistics Service, and both are used as inputs to ERS's Food Availability Data System, a data summary of the food supply chain. Economic aspects of food processors, distributors, grocery stores, and restaurants are monitored by the U.S. Department of Commerce agencies (the Census Bureau and the Bureau of Economic Analysis) and by the U.S. Department of Labor's Bureau of Labor Statistics (BLS). ERS's CFDS (the main topic of this report) aims to illuminate the consumer part of the chain, including acquisition as well as consumption. The health and well-being of the population are measured and monitored by various agencies within the U.S. Department of Health and Human Services (HHS), but without funding from USDA these agencies would lack data on food insecurity, for example. In their efforts to understand the population's health, their focus is not on the food environment or the food assistance landscape either. Hence, the responsibility for measuring and monitoring the food supply system and its impacts, including the ways it interacts with food assistance programs, falls to many different agencies. Fulfilling that responsibility requires significant collaborative efforts.

Broadly speaking, this data system for tracking sequential elements of the food supply system, focusing on consumer acquisition, is called upon to fulfill descriptive or monitoring needs, some of them essential to developing official statistics. It is also called upon to support research to examine program impact or address other causal questions. In later chapters of this report, we examine details of the current CFDS infrastructure and propose solutions for improving it. A big part of the solution involves integrating survey, administrative, proprietary commercial, and other kinds of data sources in order to exploit the strengths of each type.[2]

Key policy areas for the CFDS, which fall within the agency's purview, are headlined by:

1. **Agriculture and the food system.** How do upstream factors (such as the agroecological environment, agriculture policy, innovations in food manufacturing, new product development, and labor policy)

[2]CFDS integration of multiple data sources is discussed in detail in Chapter 2.

influence consumer food outcomes? Conversely, how are changes in consumer tastes and preferences about the food system communicated back up the supply chain?
2. **The food retail environment.** How do the location and competitiveness of small food retailers, large supermarkets and superstores, and restaurants influence consumer food outcomes? Conversely, how are changes in consumer outcomes and preferences concerning the retail environment communicated back up the demand chain to influence retail competition and location decisions?
3. **Healthfulness of U.S. diets at all income levels.** For all of these factors that influence consumer food purchase and acquisition, what is the ultimate effect on nutrition, health, chronic disease, and mortality risk?
4. **Economic determinants of consumer demand.** How do incomes and consumer preferences influence food choices and how are prices related to food choices?
5. **Food and nutrition safety net programs.** How do SNAP, WIC, school meals, the Child and Adult Care Food Program (CACFP), and other programs affect (i) food acquisition and use by people at all income levels and, in turn, (ii) the food security of and nutritionally healthy consumption by the population?

Understanding the Food Environment and Its Relationship to Health

Food choices and diet quality are influenced by the many opportunities, constraints, and challenges that consumers face in the food environment. The Centers for Disease Control and Prevention (CDC) defines the food environment to be "the physical presence of food that affects a person's diet; a person's proximity to food store locations; the distribution of food stores, food service, and any physical entity by which food may be obtained; or a connected system that allows access to food."[3]

The types of food outlets that are accessible to consumers dictate the product availability, quality, and prices those consumers face. Outlets exist across a range of types, from supermarkets to convenience stores to restaurants. A consumer's (geographical) food access reflects the proximity and types of restaurants and stores present in his or her local environment, and where retail food stores are concerned an important feature is whether a store is authorized to participate in one of the USDA food assistance programs. Food is also provided by schools, child care providers, pantries, and nursing homes, and all these can affect the food environment.

---

[3] See https://www.cdc.gov/healthyplaces/healthtopics/healthyfood/general.htm.

Within this topic area of the role the food environment plays in people's food choices, key descriptive and monitoring questions include these:

- How many people have limited access to sources of healthy and affordable foods?
- Does ease of access matter for nutritional quality of purchases?
- Where do people buy and consume food?
- How does food preparation affect food safety?
- Do food assistance programs affect these choices?

Causal impact questions (with program policy implications) include these:

- How do food store access, access to restaurants, and the larger food environment impact food choices, diet, and diet-related health?
- How do food access and regional price variation jointly affect these outcomes?
- How do consumers respond to new information and product attributes?
- How do other factors, such as income, time resources, and consumers' preferences and knowledge, affect food consumption decisions; and how have these factors and connections changed over time?
- How do food assistance programs affect these choices?

Concerning ease of access, USDA has provided mapping tools in applications such as the Healthy Food Finance Initiative and the Food Access Research Database. There has also been some debate over new SNAP stocking requirements, so these two data projects are useful for community and local planning use.

Surveys currently serve as one data source to address many of these questions. In particular, ERS's National Household Food Acquisition and Purchase Survey (FoodAPS)—described in detail in Chapter 2—generates information not captured elsewhere about spending by consumers at specific retailers as well as access to other sources of food (including food in-kind from local organizations, family, neighbors, or friends), about distance to primary food retailers, and about consumer attitudes and opinions regarding food retail access for a point in time. The central role of surveys notwithstanding, the use of both proprietary commercial data (e.g., NPD Group data on the locations of restaurants and Nielsen price data for retailers) and administrative data (e.g., from SNAP and WIC programs) is expanding rapidly as new opportunities emerge. At the same time, surveys are becoming less viable as the sole source of information for reasons of cost and quality.

Improved access to administrative and proprietary data is opening new opportunities, though it is worth noting that surveys are key sources of data covering the entire population. For example, due to survey problems with underreporting and, to a lesser extent, with over-reporting, administrative data on use of any single program are typically superior for measuring participation. However, such administrative data cannot provide data on the universe of individuals who *could* participate in a program but are instead restricted to those who have participated. Without also knowing about nonparticipants or participants in other programs, key questions about policy effects, program take-up, and impacts of programs on health and nutrition outcomes cannot be answered.

Finally, it is difficult to generate causal estimates of the effects of programs outside randomized control trials without contextual information about program rules at the state and local levels. The panel's recommendations for advancing ERS's CFDS (Chapter 4) are largely focused on survey collections, enabling linkages between survey and nonsurvey data sources, establishing and maintaining searchable policy databases, and monitoring the quality and coverage of proprietary data sources.

Supporting Program Policy and Administration for the Food and Nutrition Safety Net

Food assistance programs serve a large share of the population. At some point during a given year, about one in four Americans participate in at least one of USDA's 15 domestic food and nutrition assistance programs. As indicated in the budget figures cited at the beginning of the chapter, these programs accounted for $98.6 billion in spending in 2017—more than two-thirds of USDA's annual budget, but well below historical highs (Oliveira, 2018, p. iii). The largest of these programs in terms of spending is SNAP, which serves as the foundation for the country's nutrition safety net. While at around $6 billion annually WIC has lower expenditures than several other programs, it touches around half of all infants. Similarly, the school meals programs subsidizes a large share of meals at schools every day.

Policy makers, other stakeholders, and the public are interested in understanding the impacts of these substantial investments. This requires accurate information about program participation; the factors that affect take-up of programs among those eligible to participate; the profiles of program participants; and the food choices, nutrition, and health outcomes associated with participation. Importantly, the influence of program participation should be modeled in a way that makes it possible to study causal relationships and to allow researchers and policy makers to monitor the performance of these programs. Questions, some descriptive and some causal, that need to be regularly answered for affective administration of safety net programs include the following:

- Who participates in USDA food assistance programs? And in what ways are SNAP and low-income households similar to or different from the overall population along different dimensions? (descriptive)
- Among those who are eligible, who does not participate? (descriptive)
- Among those who do not participate, why not? Is this driven by policy or other factors? (causal)
- What are the program participation rates, both as a percentage of the relevant categorically eligible populations and as a percentage of all eligible persons? (descriptive)
- How are participation rates affected by program rules? (causal)
- What are the program entry rates, exit rates, average spell durations for cohorts of new entrants, and average spell durations for a cross-section of current participants? (descriptive)
- What is the dietary quality profile of the U.S. population? What foods do people buy, how much do they pay, where do they shop, and what is the nutritional quality of food expenditures? (descriptive)
- What is the dietary quality profile of food expenditures for SNAP participants, low-income non-SNAP participants, and higher-income non-SNAP participants? What is the profile for those people who are joint SNAP and WIC participants? For those who do not participate? And how do these programs interact with CACFP and the school meals programs in eligibility, participation, and effects? (descriptive)
- What is the dietary profile of food *intake* (rather than food expenditures) for the different groups described above, including those participating and those not participating in the different programs? (descriptive)
- How do the respective programs affect food intake? (causal)

Since most food assistance programs are funded and administered through the USDA's Food and Nutrition Services (FNS), it is natural that measuring and monitoring the impact of those programs should fall to a separate group within USDA, such as FED. For policy purposes, the causal answers to the questions listed above and below are even more important than the descriptive findings above.

Key additional causal questions exploring program impact include these:

- How do SNAP, WIC, the school meals programs, and other programs affect food spending and dietary intake?
- How do the programs affect nutrition, food security, health, and use of health care systems?

- How do food spending and food intake respond to prices, income, and program benefits in a demand-systems framework consistent with economic theory?
- How does the safety net function during economic contractions?
- Does the food assistance safety net have unintended consequences?

To answer these questions and those envisioned going forward, researchers will rely on survey, administrative, and, increasingly, proprietary commercial sources. For example, FoodAPS has been successfully used to assess food expenditure and acquisition at a point in time; the National Health and Nutrition Examination Survey (NHANES) measures food and nutrition intake; the Current Population Survey's Food Security Supplement measures food security; and the Survey of Income and Program Participation (directed by the Census Bureau) and the Panel Study of Income Dynamics (PSID, directed by faculty at the University of Michigan) produce longitudinal data that can be used to study program participation.[4] Examples of administrative sources used to help answer questions about safety net programs include FNS data on program participation that originates at the state level; state-provided individual-level data on participants' and firms' program benefits and their use; SNAP quality control data; and the WIC Participant Characteristics Data (a census of WIC participants constructed with administrative records in April of even-numbered years).

An example of contextual data that allow researchers to study causal questions about SNAP is the USDA/ERS SNAP Policy Database. Examples of proprietary data that have been used to study how people make choices about food acquisition are scanner data collected by IRI Worldwide and Nielsen on a panel of households or from a set of retailers. Analyses employing integrated or linked survey, commercial, and administrative approaches can take advantage of the wide-ranging outcome variables in surveys and the large sample sizes and geographical disaggregation of administrative data with high-frequency data from commercial sources. These combinations have also enhanced researchers' capacity to measure "small area estimates" of outcomes such as food security by county. Administrative data also provide the ability to measure participation in many of these programs with considerably less error than survey data. Commercial data provide some high-frequency data for relatively low cost, and when combined with the other two sources, can be even more useful.

In Chapter 2, we review examples of these strategies from the literature, along with the barriers they present. Barriers include sample size limitations

[4]Current data solutions and their strengths and weaknesses are described in detail in Chapter 2; panel-envisioned solutions are advanced in Chapter 4. For example, the well-known problem of misreporting program participation is discussed there.

and self-reported program participation indicators in surveys; lack of outcome variables and a corresponding measure of the population in administrative data sources; and lack of coverage and benchmarks about quality in commercial data. Recommendations (Chapter 4) focus on the following: (i) continued targeted investment in surveys; (ii) expanded coordination and access to administrative sources; (iii) expanded use and continued quality assessment of commercial data; and (iv) expanded tracking of state and local eligibility and implementation across all USDA food assistance programs, as well as tracking of stores where benefits are redeemed.

Supporting Research on the Healthfulness of U.S. Diets (at all income levels and for all types of people)

Making headway in understanding the complex links between diet, nutrition, and health outcomes is critical for informing government food policy strategies to improve a population's well-being (Duffey et al., 2010; Olson, 1999; Marshall, Burrows, and Collins, 2014). A key example is the relationship between poor diets, coupled with physical inactivity, and obesity, which is a leading cause of preventable death and disability in the United States and in many other countries. Gorski and Roberto (2015) describe the ways in which current food environments exploit biological, psychological, social, and economic vulnerabilities that encourage overeating, and they review recent public health policies to promote healthier diet patterns, including mandates, restrictions, economic incentives, marketing limits, information provision, and environmental defaults. The authors (p. 81) point out, "unhealthy diet patterns, including high intake of added sugars, trans fats, and excess sodium intake are linked with obesity, heart disease, type 2 diabetes, cancer, high blood pressure, and stroke." Yet we know little about the causal link between these policy levers and changes in long-run health outcomes such as obesity. The CFDS offers data that may provide insight into the causal links between these policy levers and diet as well as links to longer-run outcomes, and it also allows for surveillance.

The 2015–2020 Dietary Guidelines Advisory Committee report stated, "health and optimal nutrition and weight management cannot be achieved without a focus on the synergistic linkages and interactions between individuals and their environments, and understanding the different domains of food-related environmental influences" (U.S. Departments of Agriculture and Health and Human Services, 2015, p. 1).[5] Evaluation of food-related health policies to determine how well they are accomplishing their goals requires access to high-quality consumer-level panel data. While the Guidelines

[5]This advisory committee serves HHS and USDA, which jointly publish the Dietary Guidelines for Americans (Dietary Guidelines) every 5 years.

process typically uses NHANES data (which has the weakness of 24-hour recall surveys) in its analyses, rather than data generated by ERS, FoodAPS might provide alternative data that could be useful in assessing existing U.S. dietary patterns as well as adjustments that might be made to diets (again recalling the weaknesses of 24-hour-recall surveys such as NHANES).[6]

A partial list of questions about food-related health policy including diets, nutrition, obesity, and health care—some of which are causal in nature and some of which are descriptive—includes the following:

- What foods do households buy? What is the nutritional quality of the foods they acquire? What about the food they consume? How much are they willing to pay and where do they shop?
- What impact has the application of federal nutritional standards for all foods and beverages served in schools had on overweight and obesity among school-age children?
- What are the impacts of SNAP and other programs on food purchases, food consumption, diet quality, food insecurity, overweight and obesity, and other health outcomes?
- What effects have food assistance and nutritional educational programs had on the nutritional quality of diets of those served by the programs?

Data sources available to help to provide answers to these questions include nationally representative surveys as well as data from proprietary sources, which are typically not nationally representative. Key surveys for tracking food acquisition and consumption include NHANES,[7] sponsored primarily by the National Center for Health Statistics (NCHS) of CDC, which uses a dietary recall survey to collect information about food intake; the Consumer Expenditure Survey, sponsored by BLS, which collects data on expenditures for food at home and food away from home using two 1-week diary surveys; the food expenditure questions in PSID, funded by ERS; and the above-noted FoodAPS, sponsored by ERS, which collects household food expense data by asking selected households to scan their food receipts, as well through food diaries and telephone interviews.

Other nonsurvey data sources that are increasingly being used to measure food acquisition include proprietary data, such as the Consumer Network by IRI Worldwide and HomeScans by Nielsen, which provide con-

[6]The same parent department, USDA, comprises both ERS and the Center for Nutrition Policy and Promotion, which is the department's lead agency on the Dietary Guidelines for Americans.

[7]NHANES collects a wide variety of information other than food intake as well. See http:///www.cdc.gov/nchs/nhanes/about_nhanes.htm.

sumer data from a panel of volunteers, and Infoscan from IRI Worldwide, which provides scanner data from food stores. Other surveys, such as the Current Population Survey's Food Security Supplement, National Health Interview Survey (NHIS), NHANES, and PSID, all track food security.

Facilitating Answers: ERS's Data Collection Approach

Increasingly, ERS's approach to answering the types of research and policy questions described above is to emphasize an integrated mix of data sources. To address many of these major public health policy issues, research on causal effects of programs on nutrition and health outcomes is particularly important. To advance research in topic areas that fall within its purview, FED is actively engaged in developing a data collection strategy that draws on a wide variety of sources. Bringing together all these sources makes it possible to combine survey, administrative, and proprietary data on the food environment, production, processing, and food items (from retailers and restaurants) with related information on the consumers, including their nutritional intake and status, the affordability of their food purchases, and their health outcomes.

Larimore and colleagues (2018) describe three specific FED initiatives reflecting this multiple-data-source approach that were born, in part, out of recommendations from an earlier Committee on National Statistics report (NRC, 2005): (i) expanding the use of proprietary data; (ii) developing the Next Generation Data Platform; and (iii) creating an innovative consumer acquisition survey, realized as FoodAPS, which was first fielded in 2012.[8]

ERS has had extensive experience (relative to most statistical agencies) with commercial data, including acquiring it, assessing its quality, and using it to answer questions about food acquisition. For the most part, these data fall into one of three categories: proprietary retail scanner data,[9] household panel and scanner data, and food store and restaurant name and location data.[10] Retail scanner data are collected in stores during customer checkout, while household scanner data are collected using hand-held scanners provided to participating households. An advantage of scanner data (over survey data, for example) is that reading devices detect and record exactly which product is purchased and sometimes, though not always, also collect its price (Larimore et al., 2018, p. 8).;[11] Chapters 2 and 4 discuss the

[8]Information in this section is drawn from Larimore et al. (2018) and from presentations by ERS staff and others at the workshops described in Appendix A.

[9]A scanner uses a laser to read the Universal Product Code (UPC) on a store item's label.

[10]Presentation to the panel by Mary Muth, September 21, 2018.

[11]Advantages and limitations of these commercial sources are covered in detailed in Chapter 2, section 2.4.

insights that have and can be drawn from scanner data, and also issues—such as their frequent lack of critical geographic coverage or of identifiers needed to link stores across datasets—that need further attention in order to improve returns on future investments in such resources.

Commercial data have been usefully applied by ERS and other researchers to policy-oriented matters, such as identifying the composition of food purchases by WIC household versus non-WIC households (e.g., types of products, such as breakfast cereals); identifying the use of WIC benefits (by identified food items); measuring the effects of WIC program participation on food purchases; and evaluating the effects of program changes on food purchases over time.[12] However, this WIC example also suggests the value of linking administrative data to such proprietary data, if possible, because otherwise WIC use has to be inferred from self-reports or from the food item scanning records, both of which are likely to lead to measurement error.

The Next Generation Data Platform, discussed in detail in Chapter 2 (section 2.2), is a strategic partnership formed in 2012 with USDA's FNS and the Census Bureau. This joint project is a long-term effort to acquire state-level administrative data for USDA nutrition assistance programs—especially SNAP and WIC—and to make those data available for linkage to other administrative files and surveys. In this work, FNS contacts state SNAP and WIC offices to encourage them to share their USDA administrative data for the project, and the Census Bureau negotiates a data-sharing agreement that provides mutual benefits for all parties.[13] For example, one anticipated research application of the program is the ability to evaluate SNAP and WIC participation and nonparticipation by county within a state, as well as by various demographic and other variables captured in the Census Bureau's American Community Survey. These data will also permit research into how food program rules affect the take-up of programs as well as other outcomes.

As noted earlier (and as detailed in Chapter 2), FoodAPS, which was designed in collaboration with FNS, was conceived of in response to the recognized limitations of U.S. consumption and expenditure surveys. For example, dietary recall data, which are generated by food consumption surveys, are collected to learn about patterns of individual-level food consumption and about the nutrient content of foods consumed, but these data convey no information about where the foods were acquired. Consumer expenditure surveys provide information for learning about household food expenditures. Both of these traditional sources fail to provide a complete

---

[12]Muth et al. (2016) provide a full accounting of the application of commercial data, particular scanner data, to food policy research.

[13]As of mid-2017, 20 state SNAP agencies (including 39 counties in California) and 11 state WIC agencies were partners in the Next Generation Data Platform. See Prell (2018) for a summary of state-level participation.

picture of the amount and types of foods that households acquire and how those acquisitions are affected by food prices, the local food environment, and participation in USDA's food and nutrition assistance programs.

FoodAPS, which was fielded from April 2012 through January 2013, was the first nationally representative survey designed to collect comprehensive data on foods that households purchase or acquire from all sources whether obtained by money or for free. It is notable in capturing data on the way most households also tap into "non-purchased" or so-called free sources—such as food pantries and food supplied by friends and relatives as well as by employers, schools, and child care providers—to supplement their bought food, and these foods do not appear in expenditure surveys (Larimore et al., 2018, p. 9).

FoodAPS data have been used to address important policy-relevant issues with both descriptive and causal approaches. These issues include where households acquire food in a typical week, which foods they acquire, and how much they pay (Todd and Scharadin, 2016); which factors affect households' decisions about where to shop for food (Ver Ploeg et al., 2015; Ver Ploeg, Larimore, and Wilde, 2017); which household characteristics are associated with increased childhood obesity risks (Jo, 2017); how SNAP benefits are used over the course of the benefit month (Smith et al., 2016); price sensitivity among WIC households (Dong et al., 2016); and how price variation across geographic areas affects the adequacy of SNAP benefits (Basu, Wimer, and Seligman, 2016). While the acquisition data that FoodAPS provides are rich, they limit a researcher's ability to study some causal questions because the data derive from food acquisition at a single point in time.

Elsewhere on the survey front, ERS has actively expanded its portfolio by sponsoring or cosponsoring modules on surveys conducted by other agencies. Among the noteworthy modules that have been developed are the Food Security Supplement, which has been added to many surveys (see the list in Box 2.1); the Flexible Consumer Behavior Survey, a module which has been added to NHANES, conducted by NCHS; and the Eating and Health Module, which has been added to the American Time Use Survey, part of the Current Population survey conducted by BLS.

Improving researchers' access to data is another important aspect of ERS's CFDS data strategy (discussed in detail in Chapter 4). ERS collaborates with researchers in academia and with research organizations through grants and cooperative agreements. ERS has sponsored FoodAPS research by external researchers through a National Bureau of Economic Research grants program and a University of Kentucky Center for Poverty Research (UKCPR) grant program.[14] Additional research to enhance

[14]ERS also sponsored the UKCPR grant program to conduct research on NHIS and PSID.

the nation's nutrition assistance programs has been sponsored by USDA through the Tufts University/University of Connecticut Research Innovation and Development Grants in Economics Program, established to "address national objectives for improved food security and dietary quality."[15]

ERS has also broadened public access to FoodAPS by removing identifying information about survey participants and posting the edited files and documentation on the ERS Website. ERS has made confidential survey data from FoodAPS available to researchers through a secure data enclave at NORC, an independent research organization at the University of Chicago. Beyond this arrangement, the agency is working with the Census Bureau, FNS, and state partners to make confidential administrative data and linked data available through the national network of Federal Statistical Research Data Centers. Data from modules and supplements cosponsored by ERS are available through the access procedures provided by the agency that collects the data. Commercial scanner data on people and stores are available for collaborative work with ERS researchers, although (as discussed later) the commercial entities providing such data impose limitations that mean these data are not always available to those at public institutions.

1.3. CHARGE TO THE PANEL; REPORT THEMES AND STRUCTURE

In 2017, ERS's FED asked the National Academies of Sciences, Engineering, and Medicine's Committee on National Statistics (CNSTAT) to provide guidance for further development of its consumer food data system over the next decade. The mission of FED, as described to the panel,[16] is to evaluate contemporary and anticipated food policy and program objectives, as well as market trends and dynamics; to develop the necessary data and information infrastructure to examine evolving questions; and to produce the right products and information for the administration, the Congress, and the public on consumer food choice behaviors and outcomes such as nutrition and health. In support of this mission, according to its Webpage:

> FED conducts economic research and analysis on policy-relevant issues related to the food sector (food safety, food prices, and markets); consumer behavior related to food choices (food consumption, diet quality, and nutrition); and food and nutrition assistance programs (Supplemental Nutrition Assistance Program (SNAP), Women, Infants, and Children's

[15]See https://ridge.nutrition.tufts.edu/research-grants/2019.
[16]Presentation to the panel by Mark Denbaly, April 16, 2018.

Program (WIC), National School Lunch Program). Food and Economics Division also provides data and statistics on food prices, food expenditures, and the food supply chain.[17]

FED adopted guidance from an earlier report by CNSTAT (NRC, 2005) to create a blueprint for enhancing its consumer data program—a portfolio of data resources that measure the country's food and nutrition conditions and the factors that affect those conditions.

This report is intended to reconsider how FED's consumer food data collections are conceived, how it adapts over time to challenges, and how it exploits new opportunities. The testimony that the panel heard during its public meetings was striking in its portrayal of the challenges faced by traditional survey approaches, of the new opportunities (and problems to overcome) in exploiting administrative and commercial data, and of the benefits of blending all three types of data sources, that is, survey, administrative, and commercial data.

No single data source—or even single data type—can provide all the information needed to understand the food sector, including consumption, diet, and nutrition. Policy makers and researchers who rely on FED data include those within USDA as well as those in other agencies whose responsibilities are related to food outcomes, including those within HHS and the Environmental Protection Agency. Other stakeholders include state and local policy makers, food producers, food retailers, consumer groups, think tanks, nonprofit groups, and academic researchers. The multiplicity of data sources and distributed food-related responsibilities make collaborative efforts imperative for reducing duplication and gaps. In particular, the panel that produced the 2005 report (NRC, 2005) supported collaborative interagency activities to create linkages between surveys, administrative data, and other data; to develop food-related modules to be used on relevant federal surveys; and to evaluate use of proprietary data (collected, owned, and made available by commercial firms).

Aims and Focus of This Report

This report is intended to provide a blueprint for ERS's Food Economics Division for its data strategy over the next decade. ERS leadership specifically asked that the panel address the following questions:[18]

- Are the current data collected or supported by ERS delivering policy-relevant evidence that is as credible and insightful as possible?

[17] See https://www.ers.usda.gov/about-ers/agency-structure/food-economics-division-fed.
[18] Presentation to the panel by Jay Variyam, April 16, 2018.

- Is the current multiprong data approach—and particularly the balance between the use of survey, administrative, and commercial sources—the correct one, or is there a better practical use of resources?
- Given key current and emerging policy questions, which kinds of data are anticipated to become the most valuable to researchers, policy makers, and program administrators going forward?
- Should the nation have a comprehensive food acquisition survey like FoodAPS and, if so, how frequently should it be conducted? If not, what are the alternative uses of resources now used to fund this survey?
- Considering the new data opportunities made possible by the Web, by wearable devices, by mobile technologies, by apps, and by big data, which ones should ERS be considering?

Motivated by the goal to improve the data infrastructure supporting research and policy in the topic areas outlined above, the authoring panel of this report was charged with addressing the statement of task (see Box 1.1). In addressing this charge, the panel identified key questions that CFDS data are used to address. Data are needed to produce descriptive content, to serve monitoring functions, and to support causal and other kinds of policy research spanning topic areas ranging from the food environment, to informing program policy, to understanding the healthfulness of people's diets. The present report first describes the current ERS data infrastructure—which includes survey, administrative, commercial, and combined data elements—and then proposes data solutions to better answer questions that, as of now, cannot be satisfactorily addressed.

One prominent part of this charge, although certainly not the only one, is to provide guidance to ERS on directions for future iterations of the FoodAPS survey. Specifically, the panel aimed to answer these questions: Should FoodAPS be a permanent data collection effort? Is FoodAPS as currently constructed worth the investment or should it be pared back? Can FoodAPS be better combined with other administrative data? What are the alternative data investment options? Would alternative investments generate similar or greater research and policy content or not? Recommendations about the future direction of FoodAPS, formally presented in Chapter 4, include three messages: (1) a caution on costs—that USDA should note the expense of FoodAPS and be careful about not displacing other data sources and staff activities through over-investment; (2) the need to make the survey cycle predictable—if budgets permit continued investment in FoodAPS, the survey should be fielded on a consistent time interval; and (3) the importance of continued cost reduction—FoodAPS can be streamlined and its quality enhanced simultaneously through continued investment in linkage

BOX 1.1
Statement of Task

An ad hoc panel will review the Consumer Food Data System (CFDS) program for the Economic Research Service (ERS) in the U.S. Department of Agriculture (USDA) and provide guidance for its advancement over the next 10 years. Among the key components of the ERS food and nutrition data infrastructure are: the National Household Food Acquisition and Purchase Survey (FoodAPS), supplemental modules to existing federal surveys, administrative data residing in USDA and other agencies, commercial data sources, and the capacity to perform linkages across databases. The value of the CFDS program is realized from supporting research that informs high-priority current—and anticipated future—policy questions, some of which are state and locally focused (e.g., research on school lunch menus and nutrition, and on food choices of households given the distribution of retail outlets). The ultimate goal of the CFDS program is to advance understanding of the impacts of the food environment, food assistance programs, and other public health policies on a range of behaviors and outcomes related to participation in programs, food acquisition patterns and where food is obtained, dietary choices, and nutrition.

The panel will also seek to identify data gaps and to anticipate how evolving policy priorities may affect data needs. Special attention, for example, is often required to capture: expenditure and consumption information on difficult-to-survey demographic groups; information on purchases for certain categories of food (e.g., snacks, meals consumed for "free"); and acquisition, sales or volume information from some types of food outlets (e.g., food pantries, independent stores).

Accessibility of data by the user community also affects the return on public investment and is therefore an important consideration in a longer-term data infrastructure plan. The panel's recommendations should recognize the rapidly changing data landscape in which surveys have become more costly and lower-burden alternative data sources have emerged. Changing consumer food shopping modes (e.g., increased food shopping online) will likely continue to elevate the importance to researchers of nonsurvey data sources such as proprietary data and administrative data. Assessing the quality, coverage, and representativeness of these data sources will be increasingly important. Maximizing the potential of the full range of information sources by ERS and other statistical agencies will require coordination among them to avoid duplicating efforts.

As part of its information-gathering activities, the panel will conduct a series of public sessions to ascertain the views of data providers, data users, and survey experts. The panel will produce a consensus report with conclusions and recommendations.

across survey and administrative and commercial data sources, and early planning for how those data sources will be used in public use files.

The panel was also asked for guidance about building the agency's broader data infrastructure. Relevant questions here are: What is the feasibility of Web-based data collection methods? How can expanded investment in food data (e.g., UPC product dictionaries and restaurant menu databases) complement existing data resources? How can development of regional food price indices be enhanced using retail scanner data, and how can geographic components be enhanced with area-based local demographics and policy characteristics?

The process by which the panel met its charge included four open meetings in a workshop format to gather information. These meetings were intended to inform the panel as it began shaping a strategy for producing a report that fully addresses its charge. Workshop topics of interest included the current and potential use of commercial and other nongovernment, nonsurvey data sources; users' perspectives on directions for ERS's FoodAPS survey; issues with data quality; and the linking of data sources. At later meetings, researchers presented ideas for improving food and nutrition data—including the integration of commercial and administrative data—to inform key policy issues. Among the topics discussed were the following:

1. The value (and limits) of linking SNAP or other food assistance administrative data not to surveys but to other types of administrative data to provide a "universe" of people affected by the programs. Possible universe files could be provided by data such as state unemployment insurance system data on workers covered by the system; Medicaid enrollment and claims data, which would cover a large share of low-income individuals; and public K–12 education data, which would cover a large share of families with children.
2. The limits of existing survey data and suggestions about how they could be made more useful.
3. Use of data from retail loyalty-card customers and other commercial data linked to state administrative records across most public programs to analyze a wide range of questions including how SNAP benefits are spent and what evidence is needed to design a "smarter SNAP."
4. Food consumption data needs for studying the determinants of diet quality and health-related outcomes (healthy eating index scores and body mass indexes are examples of outcomes indicators).

The panel also heard from experts on the potential of data integration and linkages for policy research and the use of administrative data. Practices being developed by the statistical agencies for combining data sources were also discussed, including the Next Generation Data Platform—a Census-ERS-FNS collaboration that links SNAP (19 states and 39 counties in California participated in 2017) and WIC (11 states) data to Census survey data and administrative data. Challenges discussed included the fact that not all states have participated in the Next Generation program. Since administrative data are often missing key pieces of information necessary to produce thorough descriptive or causal analysis, linked data can resolve some missing data or measures. However, efforts to improve the quality and comprehensiveness of existing administrative data resources are an important first step. Also, administrative data are often not available for some of the most vulnerable geographic areas or communities. Finally, as recommended in Chapter 4, many researchers currently have difficulty accessing linked administrative data, and efforts are needed to broaden who is able to access such resources.

Additionally, the panel heard several presentations about data needs from those in the policy environment studying nutrition or food assistance programs and those running the programs at a more local level. A topic of particular interest was the U.S. Commission on Evidence-Based Policymaking's guidance on the importance of states making individual-level participant data from federally funded programs available for research by the Federal Statistical System. Workshop presentations are summarized in detail in Appendix B of this report.

Outline of the Report

The remainder of this report describes ERS's current consumer food data system, assesses remaining gaps for research and policy use, and outlines guidance for filling those gaps. Chapter 2 reviews the survey data sources relied on by ERS and other relevant statistical agencies and describes the purposes these data are intended to fulfill. The chapter then describes how survey sources and program administrative records have been combined to improve the accuracy and coverage of data used for statistical purposes. Next, it documents ERS's use of commercial data and its assessments of the coverage and quality of those data, along with how those multiple data sources have been combined by ERS to produce useful resources for stakeholders. In some cases, the far-ranging data sources are used to generate statistics for descriptive or monitoring purposes; in others, these sources are used for research—ideally, to better understand causality—into program impacts and into the links between food/diet and health.

In Chapter 3, data and knowledge gaps in the areas of food, nutrition, and safety net research are identified. The chapter discusses the progress made by ERS to date in modernizing data infrastructure along with those policy and research questions that remain difficult to answer with the given data options. Specific data and measurement needs for addressing these questions are described.

Chapter 4 lays out strategies to advance the CFDS infrastructure. Most of the panel's recommendations for moving ERS data forward are presented and supported here. Desirable characteristics and qualities of a consumer food data system are discussed, and then a path is laid out for development of a forward-looking research- and policy-driven data infrastructure that will necessarily require integrating different kinds of data sources—most notably, survey and administrative data. Here, FoodAPS and complementary and alternative data sources are considered. Implications for the survey component of the CFDS are discussed alongside opportunities and challenges associated with expanding the use of administrative records and commercial data sources. Finally, the chapter discusses the issues of data access and confidentiality constraints as they relate to a statistical system that is increasingly based on multiple sources of data, acknowledging that overcoming these constraints will require investment.

2

ERS's Current Consumer Food and Nutrition Data Infrastructure

The U.S. Department of Agriculture's (USDA's) Economic Research Service (ERS) is responsible for collecting information and conducting research on a broad range of policy-rich domains. One such domain is represented by the Consumer Food Data System (CFDS)—defined by the agency as its "portfolio of data resources that measure, from the perspective of a consumer, food and nutrition conditions and the factors that affect those conditions" (Larimore et al., 2018, p. 1). This portfolio of data resources is used in economic analysis by researchers within and outside ERS along with related data resources from other sources. The value of CFDS is enhanced by ERS collaborations, both within USDA (with sister agencies Food and Nutrition Services [FNS], Agricultural Research Service [ARS], Center for Nutrition Policy and Promotion [CNPP], and others) and outside USDA (with National Center for Health Statistics [NCHS], the Census Bureau, Bureau of Labor Statistics [BLS], National Cancer Institute, and others).

Figure 2.1 illustrates the data inputs to the CFDS and the data outputs that result. Lines between inputs and outputs illustrate that ERS combines multiple inputs to provide public outputs. One input to CFDS includes the administrative data from the Supplemental Nutrition Assistance Program (SNAP) and the Special Supplemental Nutrition Program for Women, Infants, and Children (WIC), two large USDA food programs. The Next Generation Data Platform was initiated by ERS in collaboration with FNS and the Census Bureau to add state-level administrative data from SNAP and WIC to the Census Bureau's Data Linkage Infrastructure, available to researchers only in a Federal Statistical Research Data Center (FSRDC), a secure data center (see Box 2.1). Other inputs to CFDS include

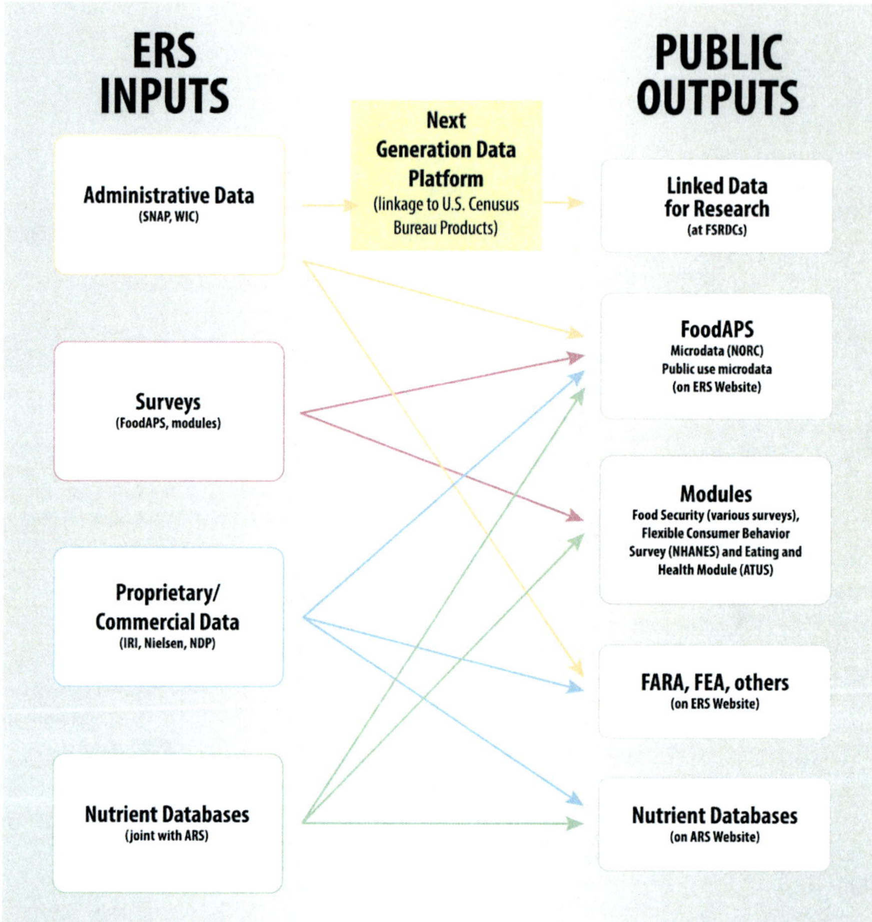

FIGURE 2.1 Overview of the Consumer Food and Nutrition Data System.
NOTES: ARS = Agricultural Research Service; ATUS = American Time Use Survey; ERS = Economic Research Service; FARA = Food Access Research Atlas; FEA = Food Environment Atlas; FoodAPS = National Household Food Acquisition and Purchase Survey; FSRDC = Federal Statistical Research Data Center; IRI = IRI Worldwide, a vendor of proprietary data; NHANES = National Health and Nutrition Examination Survey; Nielsen = a vendor of proprietary data; NORC = National Opinion Research Center at the University of Chicago, home of the NORC Data Enclave; NPD = NPD Group, a vendor of proprietary data; SNAP = Supplemental Nutrition Assistance Program; WIC = Special Supplemental Nutrition Program for Women, Infants, and Children.

data from probability sample surveys (both data from stand-alone surveys, such as Food Acquisition and Purchase Survey (FoodAPS), and data resulting from the addition of ERS modules to surveys conducted by other agencies); proprietary/commercial data (purchased from vendors); and combined data sources, such as the nutrient or food composition (crosswalk-linkage) databases (collaborative efforts among ARS, ERS, and others).

Information developed through linkage is generally more useful than the sum of its parts. Linking databases has great potential to increase their value, and it is a key ERS approach to producing public outputs. Record linkage involves finding the same entity among two or more data sources, which enables linkages over time or across programs. This is extremely valuable and, when successful, it results in an expanded database, especially if there is significant overlap between individuals in at least one of the two databases. However, record linkage can also be time-consuming and expensive to conduct, and it can be prone to error.

BOX 2.1
What Are Secure Data Centers?

Federal agencies and their contractors who collect data under a pledge of confidentiality are required by law or established policies to protect the confidentiality of individual information. Secure data centers are used to offer restricted access to confidential data. Some secure data centers also provide remote access over secure electronic lines to dedicated computers. Users must first apply, their projects must be approved by the sponsoring agency, and they must agree to terms and conditions governing the access and use of the confidential data. Any research products resulting from the data use are reviewed by the sponsoring agency to ensure that no confidential information is revealed. Currently, data from federal statistical agencies are available at either one of the **Federal Statistical Research Data Centers (FSRDCs)** or (and) the **NORC Data Enclave** (see below).

The Census Bureau established the first research data center in 1982. The Census Research Data Centers were rebranded as the FSRDCs in 2016. FSRDCs are partnerships between federal statistical agencies and leading research institutions. They are secure facilities managed by the Census Bureau and housed in partner institutions to provide secure access to a range of restricted-use microdata for statistical purposes only. The FSRDCs house data from many federal and state agencies and are available to researchers for approved projects. The Agency for Healthcare Research and Quality, the Bureau of Economic Analysis, the Bureau of Labor Statistics, the Census Bureau, and the National Center for Health Statistics are all partners in the FSRDCs and contribute data directly to them. Each agency has its own review and approval process. Other agencies also provide some of their data through the FSRDCs, especially data from surveys conducted for them by the Census Bureau. In 2019, there were 29 FSRDC locations.

continued

BOX 2.1 Continued

All RDC researchers must obtain Census Bureau Special Sworn Status—passing a moderate risk background check and swearing to protect respondent confidentiality for life—with the understanding that they may face significant financial and legal penalties under Title 13 and Title 26 for failure to do so.

For more information, see https://www.census.gov/about/adrm/fsrdc/about.html.

Since 2006, the NORC Data Enclave has provided a confidential, protected environment in which authorized researchers and power analysts can securely store, access, and analyze sensitive microdata remotely. Although larger data producers, like the Census Bureau, have sufficient economies of scale to develop advanced in-house solutions that serve the needs of external researchers, smaller agencies lack the resources to archive, curate, and disseminate the datasets they collect on their own. The NORC Data Enclave site hosts confidential data from both public and private organizations that require data security options, research computing technologies, and advanced analytics support. The enclave is located at NORC at the University of Chicago. The NORC Data Enclave currently serves more than 250 researchers and hosts confidential data for several federal agencies and foundations.

For more information, see http://www.norc.org/Research/Capabilities/Pages/data-enclave.aspx.

Record matching projects generally require access to a secure data center because of their reliance on Personally Identifiable Information (refer to Box 2.1). As noted above, the most important project undertaken by ERS in this category is its work in support of the Next Generation Data Platform, which makes state-level SNAP and WIC administrative data available for research at an FSRDC. Research projects linking the SNAP data to data from the American Community Survey have also been undertaken by ERS researchers at an FSRDC (Newman and Scherpf, 2013). FoodAPS also involved linkage with SNAP files to verify self-reported SNAP status.

Other linkage projects offer valuable insights, including those employing probabilistic matching and semantic matching. Crosswalk databases link items collected on a survey (such as quantity and type of food consumed) with important attributes (such as nutrients included and their quantities.) The nutrient databases (also called food composition databases), produced by ARS in collaboration with ERS and others, are examples of these crosswalk databases. Further development in nutrient databases are described in Poti and colleagues (2017), and Carlson and colleagues (2019) describe an additional crosswalk between the ARS data and scanner data. The geographic databases from ERS, which include the Food Access Research Atlas

(FARA) and Food Environment Atlas (FEA), are also crosswalk databases. These make use of respondent geography, such as county of residence, to link to attributes about that county, such as the percentage of households that are low-income (from the American Community Survey), or average distance from housing units to the closest food store.

ERS uses each of the input data resources in conjunction with the others to prepare public outputs. Public outputs typically include tables or spreadsheets, including crosswalk databases, graphs, maps, and public-use microdata files available on the ERS (or ARS) Website. These data products are checked by the agency to ensure that respondent confidentiality has been protected. The Office of Management and Budget's (2005) Statistical Policy Working Paper 22 describes statistical disclosure limitation techniques that are used for this purpose,[1] but there is ongoing research to develop improved methods, especially at the Census Bureau. ERS also provides confidential FoodAPS microdata files that can be accessed by the public for approved projects at the NORC Data Enclave, a secure data center where respondent confidentiality is protected (refer to Box 2.1).

Most of the data sources described here already play a central role in the current data infrastructure; others are recent innovations that do not yet have a central role but present new opportunities. An example of the latter is the Next Generation Data Platform, which is not widely known among the research community outside of government. It provides state-level administrative data on participation and benefits from SNAP and WIC, as well as on programs sponsored by other agencies, such as the Temporary Assistance for Needy Families (TANF) program and Medicare. Thanks to the Next Generation Data Platform, SNAP and WIC administrative data can be linked to Census Bureau survey data for approved projects. These data are available only to users for approved projects in a secure FSRDC. The data also incorporate Protected Identification Keys (PIKs), which support authorized users in linking individual records across these sources.

Policy and research questions drive ERS's data investment choices to maintain and advance the CFDS. Broadly speaking, CFDS products, in conjunction with data from other sources, are intended to serve descriptive and monitoring purposes and to provide inputs into causal research. Supporting causal research places greater demands on the data infrastructure than the purely descriptive function places on it. Core topics in such causal analyses may be assessed or reassessed over time. They include understanding the effects of the food environment on diet and health, understanding links between the diet and health of consumers, identifying the extent to which diets are out of balance with dietary guidelines, and measuring the effectiveness of USDA's food and nutrition assistance programs in improving outcomes.

[1]See https://www.hhs.gov/sites/default/files/spwp22.pdf.

Many of the questions in CFDS are intended to have a strong geospatial dimension. Data showing geographic variation in outcomes over time can be used to estimate causal impacts. For example, data that contain outcome measures as well as identifications of the county of birth or residence of program recipients at early ages can be used to gauge how people's exposure to different SNAP policies—that is, to the rollout over time of SNAP policies in different states or counties—affects those outcomes. Another example where fine geographic information is important is in studying how the food environment interacts with locations where program benefits are redeemed, such as grocery stores (e.g., Allcott et al., 2019).

Administrative and commercial/proprietary data have proved to be useful for revealing such geographic granularity. The Store Tracking and Redemption System (STARS)[2] from FNS (1989–2017), TDLinx from Nielsen (2004-2017), and ReCount from the NPD Group (1998–2017) have all been used to assess characteristics of the food retail environment, such as the locations and characteristics of food retailers and restaurants.[3] Descriptive information on the ways food acquisition and consumption vary based on context is important, but it is also critical to have data on outcomes across locations and time periods that reflect responses to policies over time. Such data can be used to measure how program changes and other changes in the food environment affect food acquisition, food consumption, nutrition, and health.

In the remainder of this chapter, we provide detail on ERS efforts to improve its use of alternative data sources, including surveys, administrative, proprietary/commercial, and combined data, to improve and expand its products. We also point out the collaborators who have facilitated this work. Section 2.1 describes ERS survey data initiatives and summarizes some of the other key federal surveys of importance to economic analysis of the food environment.

One key ERS initiative is FoodAPS, which is currently a stand-alone survey. This is described in the first subsection of 2.1. Another ERS survey-related innovation is the development of modules that are added to surveys conducted by other agencies. Included in that category are the Food Security Module, added to 11 surveys, the Flexible Consumer Behavior Survey, which was added to the National Health and Nutrition Examination Survey (NHANES), and the Eating and Health Module, added to the BLS American Time Use Survey. These are described in the second subsection of 2.1.

---

[2] STARS includes information about authorized SNAP retailers.

[3] See, for example, Taylor and Villas-Boas (2016a, 2016b), which examines the food store choices of low-income households; and Smith and colleagues (2016), which uses FoodAPS data to examine the "SNAP benefit cycle," in which SNAP participants exhibit higher food consumption shortly after receiving their benefits, followed by lower consumption toward the end of the benefit month.

Section 2.2 describes the administrative data for SNAP and WIC and summarizes ERS initiatives using those data, including the Next Generation Data Platform. Section 2.3 describes ERS use of proprietary data, including both food acquisition databases and store and restaurant location databases as well as the innovative products that have resulted. Included are two subsections, one describing the advantages of using proprietary data and the second describing the disadvantages. Finally, Section 2.4 describes the ARS Nutrient databases. Figure 2.1 shows these as both an input and an output because they are continually updated and expanded.

2.1. SURVEY DATA SOURCES

Data from probability sample surveys have traditionally been strong in providing representative measures of the population, but in recent years this strength has been challenged by increasing difficulties with participation rates. That in turn makes it important to note the comparatively high respondent burden and low response rates for some surveys. Survey data are also comparatively expensive to conduct on a per-observation basis. Nevertheless, survey data can provide insights into household- and person-level variables about outcomes, information that is frequently missing in administrative data.

Table 2.1 lists and summarizes the national probability sample surveys that the panel thinks have been most important to the analysis of consumer food and nutrition conditions over the past decade or more. Two of these are repeated cross-sectional surveys, two are panel surveys, and one is a longitudinal survey.[4] All collect household-level detail, demographic information, and some self-reported program participation. Of these, NHANES is the only survey to collect detailed information about food consumption on the What We Eat in America Module, sponsored by ARS. NHANES also includes extensive self-reported demographic and health-related information as well as results from a physical examination and biomarker specimens from a qualified medical practitioner. There is a long history of food consumption data both on NHANES and on the Continuing Survey of Food Intakes by Individuals (CSFII) collected by ARS in the 1980s and 1990s until 2001, when ARS and NCHS merged their respective food-related collections into NHANES.[5]

[4]Repeated cross-sectional surveys are conducted regularly, but with a new random sample selected each time. Panel surveys include at least some of the same sampled units in subsequent iterations of the survey to better capture changes over time. Longitudinal surveys collect information from only the same sampled units over time.

[5]For an overview of USDA and HHS food consumption surveys, 1936–1998, see https://www.cdc.gov/nchs/tutorials/Dietary/SurveyOrientation/DietaryDataOverview/Info1.htm.

TABLE 2.1 Summary of Federal Surveys Containing Consumer Food-Related Data

Survey Name	National Health and Nutrition Examination Survey (NHANES)	Panel Study of Income Dynamics (PSID)
Source	NCHS and ARS, conducted by a contractor	University of Michigan
Goal	To assess health and nutritional status of adults and children.	To assess the dynamic and interactive aspects of family economics, demography, and health.
Sample	Annual cross-sectional probability sample of 5,000 (achieved) households and individuals. Oversamples persons 60 and over, African Americans, and Hispanics. Current version since 2001.	Longitudinal. In 1968, a nationally representative sample of 5,000 families. Oversampled low-income. Genealogical design. In 2017 sample consisted of 10,000 families. Data collected biannually.
What It Collects	Demographic, socioeconomic, dietary, and health. The examination consists of medical, dental, and physiological measurements, as well as laboratory tests. Includes What We Eat in America Module, Food Security Module, and Flexible Consumer Behavior Survey.	Demographics, employment, income, wealth, expenditures, health, marriage, childbearing, child development, philanthropy, education, etc. Data on food at home, food away from home, total amount of Food Stamps. Food Security Module included in some interviews.
Downside	Food-intake recall method undercounts consumption. No panel data. No data on food prices or expenditures; food acquired without reimbursement.	No detail on food at home and away from home. No data on food prices, expenditures, consumption, or food acquired without reimbursement.

Consumer Expenditure Survey (CEX)	Survey of Income and Program Participation (SIPP)	National Health Interview Survey (NHIS)
BLS, conducted by the Census Bureau	Census Bureau	NCHS, collected by Census Bureau
To learn how Americans spend their money.	To assess income and program participation.	To assess health conditions.
Annual cross-sectional probability sample of 6,900 (achieved) households. Began annual collection in 1979. Has a panel component with quarterly interviews.	A series of almost quadrennial national probability-sample household panel surveys beginning in 1983. Quarterly interviews until 2014, then annual. Initial 2014 panel sample of 53,000 households.	Annual cross-sectional probability sample of expected 35,000 households (in 2019). Began in 1957. Oversamples persons 60 and over, African Americans, and Hispanics.
Expenditures, demographics, and income. Two separate surveys: the Interview Survey and the Diary Survey. The quarterly Interview Survey collects data on large and recurring expenditures with 3-month recall (rent and utilities); and the Diary Survey collects data on small, frequently purchased items, **including most food** and clothing.	Demographic characteristics, labor force participation, cash and noncash income and assets, costs for medical, shelter, child care, dependent care, and other. Occasionally includes the Food Security Module and other topical modules. Monthly event history for 4-month recall (reference period) prior to 2014. Annual reference period since.	Incidence of acute and chronic conditions, injury, physician visits, hospitalizations, and related topics using a stable core and changing modules on current health topics. Since 2011 includes adult food security module.
Limited breakdown of spending for food at home. No data on food consumption, quantities purchased, or prices.	Annual recall method likely to be subject to undercount. No data about food expenditures, consumption, or prices.	No panel data. No data on food expenditures, consumption, or prices.

Other surveys important to the analysis of the food environment include the Panel Survey of Income Dynamics (PSID), conducted by the University of Michigan with a variety of sponsors, mostly federal, including the National Science Foundation, National Institute on Aging, and National Institute of Child Health and Human Development, as well as ERS; the Consumer Expenditure Survey (CEX) sponsored by the Bureau of Labor Statistics and conducted by the Census Bureau; the Survey of Income and Program Participation (SIPP), sponsored and conducted by the Census Bureau; and the National Health Interview Survey (NHIS), sponsored by the National Center for Health Statistics and collected by the Census Bureau. However, even with this substantial history of data collection, major information gaps about food and nutrition for the U.S. population remain. The last row in Table 2.1 notes the inadequacies of each survey for purposes of monitoring food and nutrition conditions.

There have also been a large number of one-time surveys connected with particular studies, such as the large and ambitious National Food Stamp Program Survey conducted by FNS in 1996,[6] the Healthy Incentives Pilot[7] conducted by FNS in 2011–2012, and the Summer Electronic Benefit Transfer for Children study conducted by FNS in 2011–2014.[8] These surveys have yielded important insights about food security, nutrition outcomes, and poverty at national, subnational and household levels that have a wide range of policy research applications. Some of these one-off surveys have even been part of randomized controlled trials, thereby extending causal understanding of the way policy changes affect outcomes in peoples' lives. As an example, the Healthy Eating Pilot showed how subsidizing healthy purchases with SNAP can affect outcomes.

ERS initiatives in probability sample surveys include the 2012 FoodAPS and the addition of modules to surveys conducted by other agencies. These initiatives are described in the two sections below.

The National Household Food Acquisition and Purchase Survey (FoodAPS)[9]

With guidance from a National Academy of Sciences study convened by the Committee on National Statistics (NRC, 2005), ERS in partnership with FNS launched FoodAPS to close several key data gaps that had been hampering policy research. FoodAPS was intended to capture information

[6] See https://www.ers.usda.gov/topics/food-nutrition-assistance/food-assistance-data-collaborative-research-programs/national-data-sets/#NFSPS.

[7] See https://www.fns.usda.gov/snap/hip.

[8] See https://clinicaltrials.gov/ct2/show/NCT02877147.

[9] Information in this section is drawn from Larimore and colleagues (2018) and presentations made by ERS staff and others at the workshops described in Appendixes A, B, and C.

about food acquisitions from all sources (food purchases for consumption at home, food purchases for consumption away from home, and food acquired without monetary payment, by source) and to capture information about respondents' local food environment, such as distance to the nearest grocery store (by type). Another key gap was filled by using administrative data to identify actual SNAP participants.

FoodAPS was collected under the Confidential Information Protection and Statistical Efficiency Act (CIPSEA) of 2002. CIPSEA requires that the collected data be used strictly for statistical purposes and promises respondents high levels of data protection against disclosure of confidential information.[10]

FoodAPS was conducted between April 2012 and January 2013. ERS has been planning a second version of the survey, FoodAPS-2, which is described later in this subsection. FoodAPS was conducted with interviews spread over a few months, making it difficult to leverage changes in policy or the food environment to understand in a causal fashion how such changes impact food choices, food security, nutrition, or nutrition-related health outcomes

FoodAPS used a nationally representative probability sample of 4,826 households. Four target populations were of particular interest: SNAP-participating households, non-SNAP households with incomes below 100 percent of the federal poverty guideline (and therefore SNAP-eligible), non-SNAP households with incomes between 100 and 185 percent of the federal poverty guideline, and non-SNAP households with incomes above 185 percent of the federal poverty guideline (Page et al., 2019).

FoodAPS oversampled SNAP participants and other low-income households because a primary goal of the survey was to understand the food acquisition behaviors of these groups. The achieved sample included 1,581 SNAP recipient households identified from a list of then-current SNAP participants and 1,197 other low-income households. Together these two household categories made up more than half of the total sample.[11] See Box 2.2 for an overview of the FoodAPS sample design. This important use of persons known to be on SNAP as a sampling frame enabled FoodAPS to identify and recruit a sufficient number of actual SNAP recipients.

---

[10]See *Implementation Guidance for Title V of the E-Government Act, Confidential Information Protection and Statistical Efficiency Act of 2002 (CIPSEA)* at https://obamawhitehouse.archives.gov/sites/default/files/omb/assets/omb/inforeg/proposed_cispea_guidance.pdf.

[11]More precisely, FoodAPS used lists of recent SNAP participants to facilitate finding them for recruitment into the survey. Not all states provided these lists, however. Because of household mobility, changes in program participation status over time, and the absence of lists in some states, FoodAPS relied on a combination of self-reports, verification (when possible) with matching to updated state files, and the presence of observed EBT transactions in FNS's ALERT (Anti-Fraud Locator EBT Retailer Transactions) file (again, when possible) to identify the 1,581 SNAP households.

BOX 2.2
FoodAPS Sample Design

FoodAPS had four target populations of interest: SNAP participating households, non-SNAP households with incomes below 100 percent of the federal poverty guideline, non-SNAP households with incomes between 100 and 185 percent of poverty, and non-SNAP households with incomes above 185 percent of poverty. There were also four target groups: (i) the four target populations, (ii) Special Supplemental Nutrition Program for Women, Infants, and Children (WIC) household participants; (iii) metro/nonmetro classification (designated by county); and (iv) rural/nonrural classification (designated by census tract).

FoodAPS used a stratified three-stage cluster sample design. All areas in the contiguous United States had a nonzero probability of selection. The stages of sample selection included:

First Stage: 50 primary sampling units, where the primary sampling units were single counties or groups of counties. One primary sampling unit entered the sample with certainty, the others were sampled from the 947 noncertainty primary sampling units with probability proportional to size. The measure of size assigned to each primary sampling unit was a function of the estimated number of households in each target population (based on the American Community Survey's 3-year files) and the overall sampling rates of addresses within the primary sampling unit for each target population. The goals were to arrive at the target sampling rates by target population and to arrive at equal selection probabilities within groups.

Second Stage: Eight secondary sampling units (SSUs) per primary sampling unit, where the SSUs were census block groups. The sample was also drawn using probability proportional to size within the SSUs. The measure of size for selecting the SSUs was a function of the estimated number of households in each target population (based on 5-year American Community Survey files) and the overall sampling rates of addresses within SSUs for each target population.

Third Stage: The third stage of selection involved the creation of a sampling frame of addresses, stratification, and selection of addresses to serve as the screening sample for selection of households into the four target populations. The sampling frame in each SSU was based on one or more of three sources: a list of addresses from the U.S. Postal Service (USPS) Delivery Sequence File (DSF), a list of addresses of SNAP participants from 22 of the 27 state SNAP agencies in which primary sampling units were selected, or traditional field listing. In 315 SSUs, both the postal service list and the SNAP participant lists were used (this involved matching addresses on the two lists); in 71 primary sampling units only the postal service list was available; and in 14 SSUs field listing was used because neither list was available/useful. In SSUs where SNAP lists existed, the goal was equal overall probabilities for addresses in the SNAP list stratum across SSUs and primary sampling units, and equal overall probabilities for addresses in the non-SNAP stratum across SSUs. In SSUs with only the postal sequence lists or field listing, the sampling rates within SSUs were set with the goal of equal overall probabilities of selection across such SSUs.

SOURCE: Adapted by the panel based on *Review of the FoodAPS 2012 Sample Design* at https://www.ers.usda.gov/media/9068/sampledesign.pdf.

Households participating in the survey were asked to report each "food event"—a food purchase or acquisition—for a 7-day period for all household members. Additionally, FoodAPS collected data on factors that may affect household purchases and food demand, including household income, food assistance program participation, size of the household, food security, health status, food allergies and intolerances, and diet and nutrition knowledge. The survey also collected household information on major nonfood expenditures, such as rent or mortgage, public transportation, and health insurance premiums and other health-related expenses.

To provide information about health-outcome variables, FoodAPS included variables needed to calculate healthy eating index (HEI) scores and body mass index (BMI) scores (the later to capture incidence of obesity), and the Food Security Module (described in the next section). Other key covariates included self-reported SNAP and WIC participation, two administrative measures of SNAP participation, gender, race, marital status, household size, income, education, age, work, and rural tract. See Courtemanche, Denteh, and Tchernis (2019), Meyer and Mittag (2019), and Kang and Moffit (2019) for an assessment of these measures.

The inclusion of information about food acquired without monetary payment is a distinctive feature of FoodAPS. Such foods are an important food source for many families, especially low-income families. The survey collected information on foods acquired from food banks, food pantries, relatives, friends, and home gardens, as well as children's receipt of a USDA school meal (whether purchased for full or reduced price or received for free). Notwithstanding the value of this approach, FoodAPS respondents may underreport their acquisition of such food due to stigmas associated with it. The survey also captured the geographic location of food events and the distance from the household to food retailers and restaurants.

FoodAPS was pioneering in linking survey data to auxiliary data from a range of sources to reduce respondent burden and enhance capacity for data analysis. It made use of proprietary scanner data (discussed in section 2.3) to create food item descriptions and item weights, and it used SNAP administrative records (discussed in section 2.2) to create the sampling frame and allow for data quality checks on self-reported SNAP use.[12] Thirteen data sources were used to enhance the FoodAPS geography component—specifically, to fill in details about the local food environment, such as location and density of retailers, measures of access to these retailers, local food prices, and area demographics. USDA food nutrient databases (see section 2.4) were used to add micro- and macro-nutrient content and food pattern equivalents to the micro record generated by FoodAPS.

---

[12]The survey contractor matched survey records to state program files to obtain a limited amount of information, such as participation status, date and dollar amount of last issuance, and details (date, place, amount) of EBT transactions by survey households.

Due to its rich content, FoodAPS has generated a substantial body of research on nutrition assistance, dietary quality of food spending, geographic access to retailers, food acquisition away from home, food security, and food prices.[13] Data from the survey have been used in research on the nutritional quality of food purchases and acquisitions, the economics of local food retail access, evaluation of nutrition assistance programs, and other topics (Larimore et al., 2018; Page et al., 2019; Wilde and Ismail, 2018; Kirlin and Denbaly, 2017). Important descriptive and monitoring work has come out of FoodAPS, along with some work on causal questions.

FoodAPS provides data that other existing data sources do not offer. For example, NHANES identifies food intake quantities and health-related information, but it does not capture item-level food purchases or prices, and information on participation in nutrition assistance programs is self-reported by respondents. SIPP provides self-reported food assistance program participation data, with the possibility of self-reported data about Supplemental Security Income, Social Security Disability Insurance, and Old Age, Survivors and Disability Insurance, but it does not provide good data on food intake, quantities acquired, or spending. CEX collects disaggregated food spending information, but it does not have information on quantities acquired, prices, or intake. And proprietary food retail consumer panels do not include foods purchased from restaurants or food acquired without monetary payment from food pantries (Page et al., 2019).

FoodAPS combines administrative data with survey data to generate more reliable—although not perfect—estimates of program participation. Courtemanche, Denteh, and Tchernis (2019), Meyer and Mittag (2019), and Kang and Moffitt (2019) have found inconsistencies in the quality of FoodAPS appended program data across states. In a presentation to the panel for this study, Colleen Heflin laid out reasons for such inconsistencies.[14] For example, some states may maintain monthly data while others do not; and disbursement dates or caseload information may or may not be available (the papers cited above found that two states did not report disbursement dates and five states did not provide caseload data).

Nonetheless, while the measures of SNAP based on administrative records are imperfect, the findings of Courtemanche, Denteh, and Tchernis (2019) and Kang and Moffitt (2019) suggest that they are satisfactory in the sense that whatever errors exist do not seem to meaningfully affect overall conclusions (although Meyer and Mittag [2019] are more nuanced in their conclusions). Having three different measures of SNAP participation,

---

[13] A list of publications using FoodAPS data can be found at https://www.ers.usda.gov/data-products/foodaps-national-household-food-acquisition-and-purchase-survey/research-projects-and-publication.

[14] Appendix C, Meeting 3, includes a summary of this presentation.

two of which are administrative, allows for a combined measure that is surely superior to the misreported rates of self-reported program participation found in most U.S. surveys. The aforementioned research found that the biggest challenge in using FoodAPS was data missing because only 22 of 27 states agreed to provide their administrative data for use in the project, and only 20 provided their data in time to be used. To carry out research on outcomes associated with multiple program use, these papers argued for the integration of administrative data on participation in other programs, such as WIC and Medicaid, in addition to SNAP. Since Medicaid is administered by the U.S. Department of Health and Human Services (HHS), doing so would impose important additional costs and coordination issues.

USDA also invested in understanding the strengths and weaknesses of FoodAPS from the perspective of researchers and data users (Wilde and Ismail, 2018). Data users noted several strengths, compared to other data sources, such as inclusion of administrative data on participation in SNAP in participating states, oversampling of SNAP participants, completeness of food acquisition sources including both food consumed at home and food consumed away from home, and linkage of purchase events to specific retailer locations. (Unfortunately, however, distances provided for the last type of information were based on distances between retail location and home rather than distance related to the actual shopping trip). Data users also had favorable views of FoodAPS documentation and support provided by USDA.

Limitations of FoodAPS identified by researchers and data users included the long wait for the initial data release, rounds of updates to files as data cleaning continued after initial release, some missing item-level data, and (less frequently) inconsistent classification of some retail chains and implausible values for some variables. The NORC Data Enclave[15] facilitated the use of confidential data, but this involved financial costs for researchers. Moreover, a USDA confidentiality review was required before downloading output or uploading user-provided inputs (such as user-written codes), and the response time for this type of review was variable, with longer response times and greater difficulty for reviews that were in some way atypical or nonstandard.

Data users also had suggestions for improvements in data about WIC participants, food pantry use, and other topics. It was noted that the reference period in FoodAPS, which was 1 week, was short relative to the monthly cycle of SNAP purchases that prior researchers have noted (Tiehen et al., 2017; Shapiro 2005; Wilde and Ranney, 2000; Gregory and Smith, 2019; Dorfman et al., 2018). Luckily, Beatty and colleagues (2019) document that this interview period frequently spanned likely disbursal dates for SNAP and other programs. Some data users raised the possibility of eventually having some type of panel data structure in FoodAPS; while cost

[15] See http://www.norc.org/Research/Capabilities/Pages/data-enclave.aspx.

considerations may make this challenging at the household level, repeated sampling of some geographic areas in repeated rounds of the survey should be considered.

In the independent assessments of FoodAPS, several challenges were noted:

- **Response burden and response rates.** Unit nonresponse could occur at several stages (Petraglia, Kerckhove, and Krenzke, 2016), including the initial screening, initial agreement to participate, initial interview, and final interview. The weighted response rate was 41.5 percent, sufficiently low to require nonresponse analysis (Petraglia, Kerckhove, and Krenzke, 2016; Page et al., 2019).
- **Response fatigue and underreporting.** Because FoodAPS involved several distinct survey instruments over the course of more than a week, respondent fatigue and underreporting were serious concerns (Page et al., 2019). Respondent incentives helped ameliorate the problem, but independent assessments found some indication of systematic underreporting in households that might be expected to have higher respondent burden, such as larger households with more events to report (Maitland and Li, 2016).
- **Confirming the status of nutrition assistance program participation.** State administrative data files were used in FoodAPS at several stages, including for the initial sampling frame for the SNAP participant sample and, later, for checking SNAP participation status. For 20 of the 27 states that participated in FoodAPS, state SNAP Quality Control agencies provided administrative files that could be used to corroborate participation status (Page et al., 2019). An independent assessment modeled SNAP participation in the remaining seven states that did not provide data files (Maitland and Li, 2016). Once weighted participation counts from FoodAPS were compared to USDA's SNAP Quality Control files, FoodAPS appeared to underrepresent SNAP participants, particularly at the lowest income levels (Wilde and Ismail, 2018). For WIC, overall weighted participant counts in FoodAPS were lower than expected from national administrative data (Wilde and Ismail, 2018), but this is not surprising given that WIC participation was self-reported and undocumented individuals who receive WIC benefits may be reluctant to report. The facts that many sampled SNAP households were drawn from administrative SNAP records, the recall period was short, and respondents were primed to think about SNAP and food might explain why self-reports of SNAP participation were much more highly correlated with the administrative measures than in most other large surveys with self-reports of SNAP participation.

- **Measuring income.** FoodAPS included a complex battery of income questions designed to be sufficient to determine SNAP eligibility in most cases. In addition, an initial screener had a simpler set of income questions that was designed to allow triage for purposes of selecting sampled households to meet targets for SNAP participants and low-income nonparticipants. This initial screener appears to have generated underestimates of household income, leading to the misclassification of households at the time of recruitment, which complicated efforts to achieve sample-size goals even when the income variables could later be corrected based on the longer full battery of income questions (Page et al., 2019). Of course, it is hard to adequately measure gross and net income, and most surveys suffer from the challenges of using self-reports for this purpose.
- **Food identification.** One of the most complex tasks for FoodAPS was identifying individual food items acquired, both from grocery retailers and from other sources such as restaurants and food pantries (Page et al., 2019). FoodAPS respondents were given a barcode scanner, which allowed 59 percent of food-at-home items to be matched to Universal Product Code (UPC) codes, and another 16 percent of items to be matched to a project-specific, random-weight barcode sheet provided by FoodAPS to the households. Another 20 percent of items were identified based on event receipts, and 4 percent were identified from respondent descriptions. Food-away-from-home items proved even more difficult to identify than food-at-home items. Overall, the use of the hand-held scanners was valuable for many items, although a large part of the data processing burden remained in identifying the many items that could not easily be scanned and matched.

FoodAPS has been useful for providing descriptive information about how people acquire food, and it is unique in tracking food consumed both at home and away from home, including food at work, at school, and elsewhere. In general, it has been good for studying food supply and demand at a point in time. Its greatest strength is its support of systematic descriptive information about where households buy food, what they pay, and where they get food without monetary payment. Much of the value of FoodAPS stems from the way it enables researchers to compare the choices of SNAP recipients with the choices of eligible nonrecipients as well as those who are not eligible. However, it has some weaknesses in identifying eligible SNAP nonparticipants related to broad-based categorical eligibility.[16]

[16] See https://www.fns.usda.gov/snap/broad-based-categorical-eligibility.

FoodAPS also supports the study of the average distances from respondents' homes to the stores where they buy food (although not necessarily the distances of their actual shopping trips) and the study of mean expenditures by food retailer category. FoodAPS data were used to estimate a choice model and to simulate removal of shopping options; this modeling was done to estimate average and heterogeneous willingness to pay at different food retailers (e.g., regular retailers, farmers markets) and to estimate what distances people are willing to travel to acquire food in a structural model (Taylor and Villas-Boas, 2016a).

While there is a substantial and primarily descriptive literature using FoodAPS to analyze aspects of the SNAP program (Wilde and Ismail, 2018; Page et al., 2019), the first round of the survey was less successful in supporting analysis of the WIC program. This is due to the fact that WIC participation was measured using self-reports rather than administrative data, and the groups likely to be users of WIC were not oversampled. ERS plans to correct this problem in future versions of FoodAPS by using administrative data as a basis for sampling WIC participants. Assuming that frames of SNAP and WIC participants will be drawn independently from administrative data, individuals who participate in both programs may require special treatment to generate nationally representative numbers. (Note that ERS presented the proposed enhancements to FoodAPS-2 to the panel in 2018.[17] These enhancements are summarized in Box 2.3.)

In addition to information about food acquisition, a great deal has been learned from FoodAPS about the use of SNAP (cross-checked with administrative data), receipt of cash transfers, wages, salary and self-employment income, and receipt of other benefits. The largest contributions of FoodAPS to research have been about stylized facts, such as what is the average distance from home to the places people shop for food and information leveraging the random assignment of the start of the food acquisition week, which has led to studies about the SNAP cycle (Kuhn 2018; Beatty et al., 2019). Many such topics were discussed at the Symposium, "Food Access, Program Participation and Health: Research Using FoodAPS," held in 2017.[18]

The lack of panel data in FoodAPS makes it unsuitable for modeling approaches that could estimate the causal nutrition and health impacts of policy changes over time. Tracking even a subset of households over time could help meet this need, especially if the time span coincided with key policy changes. The repeated cross-sections available from FoodAPS

[17]The presentations by Thomas Krenske and Laurie May to the panel are summarized in Appendix B.

[18]Papers presented at the symposium are available in the Southern Economic Association Journal, vol. 86, no. 1 (July 2019).

BOX 2.3
FoodAPS 2: ERS Enhancements Proposed in 2018

Improvements to Sampling Plan

- Increase the effective sample size and the quality of data for the WIC domain by using WIC (as well as SNAP) administrative records in stratum design.
- Create flags to identify people who are likely to be eligible for WIC/SNAP.
- Improve the representation of children.
- Collect data year-round to make possible comparisons of summer versus winter food expenditures and food security and to evaluate shopping changes over seasons.

Improvements of Instruments to Capture or Include the Following:

- More accurate school meal program information, including degree of daily participation and participation in summer meals program.
- Food security—through use of an 18-question food security module.
- Subjective food needs, food sensitivities, health conditions (e.g., diabetes, high blood pressure, high cholesterol).
- Work schedule.
- Online food purchasing.
- Improved geographic data:
  - Travel distances to stores and restaurants
  - Geocodes for residences and food places
  - Data on work schedules to enable analysis of the effects of work hours on food purchasing and cost.

Improvements to Data Collection Procedures

- Streamline the process of collecting food acquisition information from respondents by adding look-up databases.
- Use reminders, targeted calls, and receipts to reduce underreporting.
- Replace hard-copy food logs with electronic food logs and income worksheets to reduce the response burden.
- Make efforts to achieve sample size goals and reduce nonresponse bias.
- Capture interviewer observations, implement adaptive survey design, and improve imputation to achieve sample size goals and reduce nonresponse bias.

SOURCE: Adapted and revised by the panel, based on slides presented by Thomas Krenske and Laurie May, June 14, 2018.

and FoodAPS-2 could enable researchers to examine how policy changes implemented during the time between the surveys will affect outcomes, provided the two surveys are conducted in some of the same states. For future iterations, including a subset of repeated cross-sections, would allow researchers to study the effects of state- or county-level variables, for example.

Data quality is important to all surveys. The underreporting of self-reported income, program participation, and food acquisition and food consumption plagues most surveys that collect such data, and FoodAPS is no exception. One advantage of FoodAPS is that information on SNAP participation was drawn from state administrative data for participating states, which made it possible to check self-reported versus actual participation.

At the same time, FoodAPS crowded out investments by ERS staff in other data products; for example, the Quarterly Food at Home Database has not been updated since Version-2, which covers 2004–2010. Panel members have heard that this is because of the work required to update the code to use IRI databases and that the extra resources were consumed by FoodAPS. This leads to a question as to whether the first FoodAPS was too ambitious. An in-depth discussion of recommended solutions to these shortcomings, including limiting the scope of future rounds of FoodAPS, is presented in Chapter 4.

Use of Supplemental or Specialized Modules

ERS has actively expanded its data system portfolio by creating and sponsoring or cosponsoring specialized modules that could be added to surveys conducted by other agencies.[19] This important strategy has been used to enhance old products and develop new ones. Using add-on modules also imposes less survey burden on participants than carrying out a new stand-alone survey on any given topic. Such add-ons are most useful if they permit novel descriptive measures to be presented or if they are done consistently across time and place, as this enables causal research about how outcomes are affected by policy changes or by changes in the food environment.

ERS sponsors three modules on surveys conducted by agencies other than USDA. First, the Food Security Module, fielded each year since 1995 on the Current Population Survey, tracks household food security over time. This module has also been added to many other federal surveys (listed in Box 2.4). Two more recent modules have allowed researchers to study where people buy things and how they spend time to do so: the Flexible Consumer Behavior Survey, added to NHANES, sponsored by NCHS, and the Eating and Health Module of the American Time Use Survey, sponsored by the BLS.

[19]FNS pays for some of the food security data collections (NHIS, Medical Expenditure Panel Survey, National Survey of Children's Health, PSID). Nonetheless, these projects require ERS investment in staff time to work with the agencies to obtain the food security items on the surveys, carry out data checks, recode the composite food security variables, etc.

BOX 2.4
Federal Surveys Containing the Food Security Module

American Housing Survey (AHS)
Sponsored by the Department of Housing and Urban Development. In 2015, AHS included the 10-item adult food security module with a 30-day reference period.

Current Population Survey (CPS)
Sponsored by the Bureau of Labor Statistics. From 1995 to present, CPS has included the 18-item household food security module with a 12-month reference period.

Early Childhood Longitudinal Surveys (ECLS)*
Sponsored by the National Center for Education Statistics. In 1998–1999 (ECLS-K), 2001 (ECLS-B), and 2010–2011 (ECLS-K), ECLS has included the 18-item household food security module with a 12-month reference period.

Medical Expenditure Panel Survey (MEPS)
Sponsored by the Agency for Healthcare Research and Quality. Since 2016, MEPS has included the 10-item adult food security module.

National Health and Nutrition Examination Survey (NHANES)
Sponsored by the National Center for Health Statistics. Since 1999, NHANES has included the 18-item household food security module with a 12-month reference period.

National Household Food Acquisition and Purchase Survey (FoodAPS)
Sponsored by the Economic Research Service and Food and Nutrition Service. In 2012–2013, FoodAPS included the 10-item adult food security module with a 30-day reference period.

National Health Interview Survey (NHIS)
Sponsored by the National Center for Health Statistics. Since 2011, NHIS has included the 10-item adult food security module with a 30-day reference period.

National Survey of Children's Health (NSCH)
Sponsored by the Health Resources and Services Administration, Maternal and Child Health Bureau. Since 2016, NSCH has included a food insufficiency item.

Panel Study of Income Dynamics (PSID)
Sponsored by the National Science Foundation. PSID included the 18-item household food security module with 12-month reference period in 1999, 2001, 2003, 2015, and 2017. In 1997 and 2014, it included a Child Development Supplement.

continued

BOX 2.4 Continued

Survey of Income and Program Participation (SIPP)
Sponsored by the Census Bureau. In 2001 (wave 8), 2004 (wave 5), 2008 (waves 6 and 9), and 2014 (waves 1, 2, and 3), SIPP included a nonstandard five-adult-question module with a 4-month reference period. The 2014 panel used a six-item short-form module.

Survey of Program Dynamics (SPD)
Sponsored by the Census Bureau. In 1998–2002, SPD included the 18-item household food security module with a 12-month reference period.

---

*For the ELSC, K designates that the original sample was drawn from kindergarten children, and B designates that the original sample started at birth.

SOURCE: Available: https://www.ers.usda.gov/data-products/food-security-in-the-united-states/documentation.

The Food Security Module

The Food Security Module was developed in response to the National Nutrition Monitoring and Related Research Act, passed by Congress in 1990 (PL101-445), which led to the development of a 10-year plan for assessing the dietary and nutritional status of the U.S. population (NRC and Institute of Medicine, 2013, p. 7). The Food Security Measurement Project developed and tested the food security module survey questions, which was first fielded with the December Current Population Survey (CPS) in 1995. Hamilton and colleagues (1997) reported the first of the national prevalence estimates for food insecurity and hunger. A key innovation in the 1990s, the Food Security Module improved on previous unscientific generalizations about hunger, replacing them with a monitoring data source akin to the poverty rate and unemployment rate.

Adding the food security module to many federal sources has helped to make the food security measurement and research program a success. It is also worth noting that ERS's food security measurement and research program has become a model for other agencies. For example, the U.S. Department of Housing and Urban Development (HUD) borrowed from the ERS experience by creating and implementing a housing security module. ERS also continues to collaborate across federal agencies to institutionalize food security as a key measure of well-being—for example, in the indicators for America's Children and the goals for the Healthy People Program.

The answers to the survey questions in the Food Security Module lead to categorizing a household as either *food-secure* or *food-insecure*. Being food-insecure means being unable, at some time during the year, to provide adequate food for one or more household members due to a lack of resources. Another household categorization is *very low food security*, meaning the normal eating patterns of some household members were disrupted at times during the year and their food intake was reduced below levels they considered appropriate. Evidence suggests that while there may be a subjective component to these measures, they correlate with other measures of hardship and poor nutrition (Gunderson and Ribar, 2011; Bhattacharya, Currie, and Haider, 2004).

The advantage of having a wide range of surveys with the food security module is that together they provide the ability to correlate food security with a variety of other characteristics, depending on the focus of the specific survey. In addition, by tracking food insecurity in various settings, researchers can show how policy changes affect food insecurity as well as a host of other income sources, other measures of program participation, and other health, human capital, and economic outcomes. The long (since 1995) annual history of the food security module with the CPS makes it most useful for looking at the effects of policies. The NHANES data are most useful for cross-checking how food security is related to food intake, program participation, and objective measures of health. The food security module has also been included on numerous nonfederal surveys.

The federal government's experience with food security measures on surveys has served to illuminate household-level experience with episodes or symptoms of food-related hardship, such as cutting or skipping meals or going a whole day without food because there was not enough money for food. The module has supported *monitoring* food security trends and contributed to *causal* studies of program evaluations by including appropriate covariates for use with econometric modeling techniques. Descriptive and monitoring research topics have included, for example, the relationships between disability and food security, between medical hardship (e.g., medication underuse) and food security, between chronic disease and food security, and between kinds of disability and food insecurity. Gundersen and Ziliak (2008) provide a comprehensive review of food security research.

A number of references examine the causal relationship between food program participation and food insecurity. Focusing on recent papers from the past few years that examine the effects of SNAP, we summarize the following: Yen and colleagues (2008) used an instrumental- variables approach with the National Food Stamp Program Survey to suggest that SNAP participation reduces the severity of food insecurity; Gundersen and colleagues (2017) used partial identification models with SIPP data to find that SNAP reduces the prevalence of food insecurity in households with children; and Swann and colleagues (2017) used data from SIPP in a bivariate probit model to explore the relationship between food insecurity, the household's history during the previous year, and SNAP participation. The results indicate that negative income shocks, moves, and both increases and decreases in household size increase the probability of being food insecure, while SNAP participation is estimated to reduce the probability of being food insecure. Arteaga and Heflin (2014) used variation in state kindergarten eligibility dates to explore the protective effects of national school lunch program participation on household food security among households with a kindergarten-age child in the Early Childhood Longitudinal Study—Birth cohort (ECLS-B), showing support for the contention that the National School Lunch Program reduces food insecurity; and Schmidt et al (2016) found that among nonimmigrant, low-income single-parent families, $1,000 in potential cash or food benefits from a safety net program reduces the incidence of food insecurity.

Of course, the module has limitations. The quality of its resulting data hinges on the ability of households to accurately report assessments that are somewhat subjective. For some research questions, the limitations stemming from small sample sizes are exacerbated by the rare nature of some of the items of interest, such as very low food security. Questions have been raised about how the item response theory models, including the Rasch model, were used to establish the scaling of the module's questions (NRC, 2006; Wilde, 2004). For studies of policy impact, a problem arises because these surveys have a reference time period, typically annual, that does not match well with administrative data reference periods, which are frequently monthly.

The Flexible Consumer Behavior Survey (FCBS)

FCBS has been fielded as a module on NHANES since 2007. The module supplements the NHANES dietary and health measures with economic information (income, assets, food expenditures) and self-reported information on participation in food assistance programs (SNAP and WIC). It also contains a flexible set of questions that provide information on dietary habits and behaviors, which is useful for linkage to food intake and nutrient data. The module is designed to change according to proposed or current policy climates—to continue providing timely national data to inform food and nutrition policy-making decisions.

This has allowed NHANES data to be used, for example, in high-profile studies that compare outcomes for SNAP participants, low-income nonparticipants, and higher-income nonparticipants, although it is likely that SNAP participation is underreported. FCBS has also collected information on the use of packaged food product labeling, self-assessed diet quality, diet attitudes and behaviors, awareness of MyPlate,[20] knowledge about calorie

[20] See https://www.choosemyplate.gov.

intake needed to maintain current weight, and use of restaurant nutrition labeling when dining out. Data from the module may be supplemented with American Community Survey data on demographic characteristics and local food policy through restricted-use geographic identifiers. A key innovation has been to link food economics, food consumption, and health outcome variables in NHANES, making it possible to conduct research to determine how food security is associated with objective health measures.

One of the primary objectives of adding FCBS to NHANES is to provide national data on both health variables and consumer use of food policy initiatives (such as packaged food product or restaurant menu labeling) to evaluate the impact of federal regulations.[21] However, to estimate policy impacts it is necessary to examine repeated measures of outcomes before and after policy changes within the same locations, and this is difficult to achieve with NHANES because the survey does not usually revisit the same geography and is very unlikely to revisit the same persons.

The Eating and Health Module (EHM)

EHM is a supplement to the BLS's American Time Use Survey (ATUS) that has been fielded twice, from 2006 to 2008 and again from 2014 to 2016. It is cosponsored by ERS, FNS, and the National Cancer Institute. The objectives of this module were to collect data to analyze relationships among time use, eating behavior, and obesity as well as time-use patterns of important subpopulations such as SNAP and WIC participants, grocery shoppers, and meal preparers. The module collects information on eating patterns, grocery shopping preferences, fast food purchases, meal preparation, food safety practices, general health, height and weight, physical activity, and income (Restrepo and Zeballos, 2019; Zeballos, Todd, and Restrepo, 2019). Although these data allow for a useful assessment of effects of policy change or environment change on changes in outcomes, as with other modules their value is limited by the fact that they use self-reports of program participation.

Use of ATUS is motivated by the need for information on how individuals decide to make use of their 24 hours each day, specifically in their decisions that carry short- and long-run implications for their income and earnings, their health, and other aspects of well-being. Understanding time-use patterns can provide insight into economic behaviors associated with eating patterns as well as the diet and health status of individuals. EHM

[21]Restrepo, Minor, and Peckham (2018), for example, show that restaurant menu label users consume fewer daily calories than do consumers who notice but do not use the menu labels to decide what to order in restaurants, https://www.ers.usda.gov/publications/pub-details/?pubid=88530.

data facilitate understanding whether participants in food and nutrition assistance programs face different time constraints than nonparticipants face, thereby informing the design of food assistance and nutrition policies and programs.

An innovative investment that ERS made in EHM was to include time spent eating (while watching TV, for example) among the secondary activities it surveyed. By doing this, EHM paints a fuller picture of how much time Americans spend eating. In a recent report, Zeballos, Todd, and Restrepo (2019) compare the number and timing of eating occasions reported in the 2014–2016 ATUS-EHM to the information reported in the dietary intake component of the 2013–2016 NHANES, which is considered to contain the best available data for estimating average daily dietary intake among the U.S. population. Their findings show that the core ATUS captures only a small share of all daily eating occasions. EHM helps to reduce—but does not eliminate—the gap in the estimated number of total daily eating occasions between ATUS and NHANES.

As mentioned above, EHM collects information on SNAP and WIC participation with the intent to shed light on time use in food-related activities among these groups. This is important, since there is an ongoing debate about whether the SNAP benefit is adequate, a debate that appears to center on claims about participants' needs for more food spending for processed or prepared foods due to time constraints on home cooking.[22] A recent report shows that SNAP participants waited 6.6 minutes longer between primary eating and drinking events than non-SNAP participants did. When looking at food-related activities, the report shows that on an average day in 2014–2016, non-SNAP participants, including low-income non-SNAP participants, spent less time in food preparation and food-related clean-up than SNAP participants. The report also finds that non-SNAP participants spent 36.4 percent more time purchasing nongrocery food than SNAP participants (Anekwe and Zeballos, 2019).

Finally, time use in connection with topics such as geographic access to retailers is also of interest. As with other data sources, EHM has offered an innovation, but more research is needed to better integrate it into research programs in a way that taps into its potential for policy use.

2.2. ADMINISTRATIVE DATA SOURCES

Administrative data are collected by government agencies (state, federal, or local) for purposes of administering a program. Administrative datasets may consist of individual or household applications to participate in a program or denials of eligibility. They may cover information on the

[22] See Ziliak (2016) for a discussion of the adequacy of SNAP benefits.

distribution of benefits, information on the use of benefits, or information used to assess program quality. Many of the descriptive, monitoring, and program evaluation goals discussed in this report have been well served by expanded use of administrative data residing within USDA (Larimore et al., 2018).[23] Administrative data writ large have been used for a wide range of quasi-experimental and observational studies and are particularly useful for answering questions about a program's impacts. As noted by Prell (2016):

> Administrative data contain complete and reliable information on who participates in a program, how long he or she participated, and the amount of benefits received. In addition, because administrative data have already been collected to operate the program, a re-use of the data for statistical purposes does not incur the cost of launching a new survey to collect comparable data. Linking administrative data with data from large, nationally representative Federal surveys leverages the strengths of the two data sources, gaining results that could not be obtained using either source separately.[24]

The virtues and shortcomings of administrative data for studying program trends and impacts—whether examined on their own or used to supplement survey data—are well known.[25] For example, while these data can identify individuals receiving program benefits, they cannot on their own identify those who are eligible for program benefits but did not apply. So, while they allow researchers to study program trends, they cannot be used on a stand-alone basis to study take-up or program effects. They do offer the potential to study program effects when they are linked to population data in order to study the eligible population for programs. But not all participants can be identified from administrative data with the PIKs, which allow them to be linked to Census Bureau survey and administrative data.

Participation dynamics and intensity can be depicted accurately and in more detail with administrative data than would be possible with survey data alone, because the measurement error found in self-reports of program participation on surveys can be avoided and benefit receipts can be observed directly. However, data on the set of people who could participate in a

---

[23]The U.S. Office of Management and Budget defines administrative data as data collected by government entities for program administration, regulatory, or law enforcement purpose. They include such records as employment and earnings information on state unemployment insurance records, information reported on federal tax forms, Social Security earnings and benefits, medical conditions and payments made for services from Medicare and Medicaid records, and food assistance program benefits (U.S. Office of Management and Budget, 2014).

[24]See https://www.ers.usda.gov/amber-waves/2016/november/illuminating-snap-performance-using-the-power-of-administrative.

[25]These strengths and weaknesses are well summarized in Prell (2016), which assesses SNAP performance using the power of administrative data.

program but do not—those eligible for SNAP, for example—are crucial for modeling take-up of programs, a necessary prerequisite for studying how programs affect health and nutrition outcomes in a causal sense.

For ERS, the most significant administrative data are those developed to support the USDA's SNAP and WIC programs, in part because obtaining data on the school meals program (also large programs) is even more complicated than obtaining data on SNAP and WIC, given that eligibility for the school meals program is determined by individual school districts. Informing food and nutrition program policy is a particularly important part of the CFDS mandate. For expensive programs such as SNAP, WIC, and school meals programs, it is critical to have reliable evidence quantifying the gains in improving food security as well as minimizing health issues such as obesity. The completeness and accuracy of information on the *program participant population* are known strengths of administrative data, although recent evidence from FoodAPS suggests that self-reports and administrative data on food program participation are similarly correlated with expenditure and disbursal data.[26]

The administrative data available for SNAP vary by state but can include state-level participant information, including components of income necessary for determining eligibility for SNAP, data on benefits by month, program participants' mailing and physical addresses, and likely locations where their benefits were used. They also include SNAP quality control data, which is a sample of applicants' data on inputs to the eligibility determination process and STARS, which has information on stores in the SNAP program (and those disqualified or investigated for potential fraud) as well as on program benefit redemption. WIC data can include state-level participant information as well as data on stores participating in WIC and on redemptions. The Integrity Profile (TIP) presents a summary of authorized food vendors disallowed from the program because of program violations. WIC also compiles data from the universe of WIC recipients in April of even-numbered years (WIC PC data).

SNAP and WIC are state-administered programs, and there are differences among states. This requires researchers to understand the details of the programs as administered in each state. ERS has compiled the SNAP policy database[27] for the purpose of assisting researchers with this, providing details on SNAP policies in each state over time. This database is a key resource for causal research on SNAP. Using integrated or linked survey and administrative data approaches, researchers have used the SNAP

[26]Several papers using FoodAPS, which combined administrative data from several sources with acquisition data and self-reports of SNAP participation, showed that survey data and administrative data from multiple sources had similar levels of discord (e.g., Courtemanche, Denteh, and Tchernis, 2019; Kang and Moffitt, 2019; Meyer and Mittag, 2019).

[27]See https://www.ers.usda.gov/data-products/snap-policy-data-sets.

policy database as a source of instruments for estimating program impacts using the Instrumental Variable estimation method.[28] While it is recent, ERS has also created a dataset of the timing of SNAP disbursals, which also offers the promise to provide causal evidence.

Challenges in using administrative data in conjunction with other data sources, such as surveys, for analysis include the fact that definitions of variables may be different and that the populations represented may not overlap. Income may be measured relative to different time periods (e.g., monthly versus annual), households may be defined differently (e.g., those who are living in the home versus those who are sharing expenses, including meals). Surveys often provide data on the U.S. population that lives in households, but they are unlikely to include the homeless, those who live on military bases, or those who live in group quarters.

In research with longitudinal data where the unit of analysis is defined by geography (such as a state, county, or city) at a point in time (such as a year), it is common for some of the variables to be drawn from administrative sources and others to be drawn from survey sources. An archetypal example is the large literature on whether SNAP policy changes and the unemployment rate affect SNAP participation (e.g., Kabbani and Wilde 2003; Ganong and Liebman, 2018). Administrative data can be linked at the household level with survey data to correct or improve certain variables, such as SNAP participation. This was done in part in FoodAPS. One challenge is that data are available only for states that chose to participate by providing their administrative data. There are great opportunities for enhancing use of administrative data to better understand topics such as program participation—these are explored in Chapter 4.

ERS initiatives in the use of administrative records include the Next Generation Data Platform as well as FoodAPS. For FoodAPS (as described in section 2.1) state-level SNAP participant lists (where available) were used as part of the sampling frame; current SNAP population lists were linked to respondent data to verify self-reports of SNAP participation for those selected into the sample from a non-SNAP stratum; and linkage with STARS was used to estimate the distance from each respondent's home to an authorized SNAP retailer.

The Next Generation Data Platform

Much of the progress in the use of administrative data in the federal statistical system is accomplished through the Census Bureau's authority to collect and use administrative records. Title 13 of the U.S. Code established the Census Bureau's legal authorities for collecting, accessing, and protect-

---

[28]See, for example, Rigdon and colleagues (2017); Miller and Morrissey (2017).

ing information about the nation's population and economy. It specifies that the Census Bureau should acquire and utilize records to the greatest extent possible (§ 6); engage in reimbursable studies and joint statistical projects (§ 8); and protect confidential individual and establishment data, limiting data access to statistical uses (§ 9). Title 13 also authorizes the swearing in of researchers to assist the Census Bureau to achieve its mission (§ 23).

Applications of administrative records for use in Census and survey operations have been developed for purposes of imputation, evaluating coverage, and sampling frame improvement. Under Title 13 authority, multiple data sources have also been linked using the Census Bureau's Data Linkage Infrastructure to create new statistical products that enable innovative social science research. For information about nonprogram participants, researchers often turn to probability sample survey sources, such as the Census Bureau's American Community Survey.

In 2012, ERS and FNS formed a strategic partnership with the Census Bureau called the Next Generation Data Platform. This joint project is a long-term effort to acquire state-level administrative data for USDA nutrition assistance programs, especially SNAP and WIC, and to make those data available for linkage to administrative files from other agencies and to surveys conducted by the Census Bureau, already available in the Census Bureau's Data Linkage Infrastructure. FNS has contacted state SNAP and WIC offices to encourage them to share their USDA administrative data for this project, and the Census Bureau has then contacted those offices to solicit their interest and participation. As of mid-2017, 19 SNAP agencies and 39 counties in California and 11 WIC agencies had agreements to participate in the Next Generation Data Platform. Reaching agreements with states to share confidential administrative data with the Census Bureau is a long-term effort, requiring that a separate agreement be signed by each state. Some states are concerned about unauthorized access if they share data, despite strong security and confidentiality protections at the Census Bureau. The costs associated with preparing the data and its documentation for Census use are also deterrents, although Census has offered to offset such financial burdens. Finally, some states fear reputational harm if their practices and results look less favorable than those of neighboring states in comparison studies.

When such data are available in the Next Generation Data Platform, they will be linkable to survey data collected by the Census Bureau, as well as administrative data from non-USDA sources, which include 17 state TANF agencies, the Veterans Administration (VA), HUD, and HHS (Medicare and Medicaid).[29] The resulting combined data are available to sworn

[29]Drawn from Larimore and colleagues (2018, p. 10). For additional details about the Next Generation Data Platform and its application to food assistance research, see https://www.usda.gov/media/blog/2018/01/05/collaboration-across-agencies-supports-food-assistance-research. Also see Prell (2018) for a summary of state-level participation.

Census Bureau agents for use in analysis at approved FSRDCs, provided their work has been approved as serving Census Bureau purposes.

One of the benefits of this program to USDA was anticipated to be the ability to evaluate SNAP and WIC participation and nonparticipation by county within a state, as well as by various demographic and other data from the American Community Survey, a large probability sample survey of households conducted by the Census Bureau. ERS researchers Newman and Scherpf (2013) accomplished this, linking SNAP participation data to the American Community Survey and developing a measure of SNAP participation rates and SNAP access rates for state-level geographic regions. They presented their data findings for Texas. Using the same methodology, the Census Bureau produced a visualization for New York State that was made available in 2017.[30]

This joint project addresses questions including: What types of people are likely to be eligible? Of those likely to be eligible, what types are likely to participate? How do caseloads, entries into, and exits out of the program change over time? And, how do the answers to these questions differ across counties? Notably, none of these questions satisfies the burden of providing causal answers, but increased access to data holds the promise to do so.

As noted above, often the greatest value from administrative data is created when they are blended with survey data. The Next Generation Data Platform enables linking of administrative and survey data to improve USDA models of SNAP eligibility and participation rates. Through this collaboration, program administrative records, while imperfect, have been found to accurately reflect information about participants. These sorts of linked data are also being used by a variety of researchers—primarily those internally based at the Census Bureau—to study underreporting of programs and errors in poverty measurement caused by underreporting. The American Community Survey also adds value by including annual income data to model SNAP eligibility, as well as demographic information, so that it is possible to compare the group estimated to be eligible with that estimated to be ineligible. Broader access to these data and information about what is included in them would allow an expansion of this kind of research.

One of the promises of the Next Generation Data Platform is the potential for analysis of linkages of survey data to a number of different administrative datasets. For example, with such a linked dataset, researchers could also learn about interaction effects associated with multiple program participation, such as by comparing those participating in SNAP alone, those in SNAP plus Medicaid, those in SNAP plus TANF, and those in SNAP plus unemployment insurance. One of the challenges in using the Census Data

[30]The visualization is available at https://www.census.gov/library/visualizations/interactive/snap-profiles.html.

Linkage Infrastructure is that researchers must apply to use a FSRDC and demonstrate how their work would serve a Census Bureau purpose.

2.3. PROPRIETARY COMMERCIAL DATA SOURCES

Proprietary data are collected, owned, and made available by commercial firms. To date, ERS has acquired and used commercial/proprietary data that fall into one of three categories: retail scanner data, household panel and scanner data, and food store and restaurant data.[31] Specific companies providing these data to ERS are listed in Box 2.5. One of the challenges with the use of any outside data source is understanding its quality and coverage, key to understanding how the data can best be used. ERS has actively evaluated the quality of proprietary/commercial databases and their fitness for use. Following are the results of that evaluation, along with descriptions of the products.

Retail Scanner Data

Store scanner data capture transactions for purchased products with a Universal Product Code (UPC) on their labels, as well as random-weight products (e.g., fruits and vegetables that are weighed). In so doing, scanner devices can detect and record exactly which products are purchased, the number of items, total dollars spent after discounts (if any), and total gross amount (before discount). As a consequence, researchers can infer the average price paid as the ratio between dollars spent and units purchased, since many retailers do not share individual-level purchase prices with the data aggregators (Nielsen and IRI) but prefer to share average prices within a store or across geographic areas. Of course, this means the price data are not individual prices but are averages, and this may reduce their usefulness for research. InfoScan retail scanner data from the years 2008 through 2017 have been purchased and used by ERS. According to Muth and colleagues (2016), InfoScan captures weekly food sales data from 48,000-plus stores that generate more than 6.6 billion observations per year on expenditures and quantities of UPC and random-weight food products, covering 20 percent of all store locations and 50 percent of total food sales.

Data that ERS has purchased from InfoScan include sales data from individual stores or retailer marketing areas, which represent an unprojected (unweighted) subset of total store data.[32]

---

[31] Mary Muth presentation to the panel. See Appendix C for a summary.

[32] From the perspective of the firms IRI and Nielsen, store data are seen as a census. Whether or not this is accurate, their methods do not treat these sales data as a sample. IRI data available to ERS include only those stores that have agreed to share their data. This is an obvious research limitation (see Appendix B summary of the presentation by Okrent). Infoscan, for example, does not include all large retailers (including Costco).

BOX 2.5
Proprietary Data Sources Used by ERS Through 2018

Retail Scanner Data

- *InfoScan, IRI Worldwide* (2007–2017): Retail scanner data. Includes product label data.

Household Panel and Scanner Data

- *Consumer Network, IRI Worldwide* (2008–2017): Household panel data and household scanner data. Also includes *MedProfiler* and *RXPulse* (household health surveys).
- *Homescan, Nielsen* (1998–2010): Household panel data, used in the Quarterly Food at Home Database.

Names and Locations of Food Stores and Restaurants

- *TDLinx, Nielsen* (2004–2017): Names and geospatial locations of food stores in the United States with sales greater than $1 million, used in Food Access Research Atlas and Food Environment Atlas.
- *ReCount, NPD Group* (1998–2017): Locations and characteristics of restaurants, used in Food Access Research Atlas and Food Environment Atlas.
- *InfoScan, IRI Worldwide* (2007–2017): Retail scanner data. The retail data include store information, including store name and corporate parent, address, and retail outlet type (i.e., grocery, convenience, dollar, drug, liquor, mass merchandiser, and club stores).

Private retailers and manufacturers have a long history of collecting consumer data, often for market research purposes, and the value of these data is being extended to consumer food and health research. Granularity is among the strengths of scanner data that motivated ERS to purchase them.[33] InfoScan data have become more and more detailed over time; these data are currently available for more than 1 million items identified at the individual UPC level, to which descriptions and attributes are attached, providing information about hundreds of product characteristics (e.g., brand, size, weight, type of packaging). Food price data can be pinpointed geographically to individual stores or market areas (except that some price data are averages reported by retailers), and the data are often available on a weekly basis, with the caveats mentioned above. Such information would be difficult or expensive to obtain in any other way.[34] At the same time, these data are collected for marketing or other purposes, are not nationally

[33] See presentation to the panel by Levin and Schweitzer summarized in Appendix A.
[34] Larimore and colleagues (2018, pp. 6–7).

representative, and are not well documented, and store coverage is not equal across all geographic areas.[35]

Infoscan also includes data that originate on product labels.[36] Information on calories, nutrient quantities, daily values, serving size, product claims, and (sometimes) ingredient lists can be culled from label data and attached to data on purchases. Such information allows researchers to examine health- and nutrition-related claims about products acquired—such as, that they are gluten-free, or made from whole grain, or organic, or preservative-free, or hormone- free. With the Purchase to Plate Crosswalk,[37] product label data also allows researchers to study the healthfulness of purchases, looking at nutrients or indexes such as the healthy eating index, which measures how healthy a group of foods is per 1,000 calories. (Of course, this approach may miss food waste, and it does not measure the calories consumed.)

Household Panel and Scanner Data

The second category of commercial information is household panel and scanner data. The National Consumer Panel, a joint venture by Nielsen and IRI, is used by both these firms in their household panel data products. It comprises more than 120,000 households, which provide information on their demographic characteristics in addition to food purchase information.[38] Around half of these households provide sufficient purchase data to be included in the IRI statistical panel.[39] The same households can participate in the panel every year.

Unlike retail scanner data collected at check-out, household scanner data are collected using hand-held scanning devices provided to participating households or using a mobile cellphone app. In this way, purchases can be captured for the panel of households. Again, this source includes products with barcodes and, for a portion of the panel, random-weight products. Data obtained by ERS represent the entire panel, both static households (with weights) and non-static households (without weights). The weights are created by IRI/Nielsen to make the demographics of the

[35] Mary Muth presentation to the panel (see Appendix C for a summary).

[36] Initially, these data were available as part of USDA's Gladson UPC Information Database. See https://data.nal.usda.gov/dataset/gladson-gladson-upc-information-database.

[37] The "crosswalk" uses "a combination of semantic, probabilistic, and manual matching techniques to establish a purchase-to-plate crosswalk between the 2013 IRI scanner data and the 2011–2012 USDA nutrient databases" (Carlson et al., 2019).

[38] Households self-select to participate in commercial panels, and low-income households are underrepresented.

[39] Weekly food purchase data from these households generate 72+ million food product observations from 65 metropolitan statistical areas and 8 nonmarket areas.

panel match those of the geographic area where the households live. The household data contain geographic information, including the ZIP Code and Census block indicating where each household is located (for IRI) or the three-digit ZIP Code prefix (for Nielsen). This allows researchers to append food environment information from other datasets to household panel data to look at questions about food environment or macroeconomic conditions on household purchasing patterns. Unfortunately, the exact prices paid by the household are not available for all transactions, because often IRI and Nielsen substitute averages across time, space, or chain for retailer store data.

Geospatial Information on Food Stores and Restaurants

The third type of commercial data used by ERS provides geospatial information on food stores and restaurants. ERS has made use of Nielsen's TDLinx, (2004–2017), NPD Group's ReCount (1998–2017), and IRI's InfoScan, summarized above under retail scanner data. The InfoScan retail data also include store information, including store name and corporate parent, address, and retail outlet type (i.e., grocery, convenience, dollar, drug, liquor, mass merchandiser, and club stores).[40]

TDLinx provides names and geospatial locations of food stores in the United States with sales greater than $1 million. The database is designed to provide universal coverage of grocery, club, convenience, and small-format food-selling stores, although in practice not every unit in the universe may be included. TDLinx comprises two broad retail channels, namely the grocery and convenience channels, and 10 narrower subchannels. In addition to store name, the database includes store address, geocodes, channel and subchannel, chain status, parent company name, sales volume, square footage, number of checkouts, number of employees, and indicators of sales of specific non-food items (e.g., gas, pharmacy, liquor).

ReCount is designed to cover nearly the whole universe of brick-and-mortar food-away-from-home establishments operating in the United States and includes their names and characteristics. In 2018, this included 650,000 restaurants, 130,000 convenience stores, and 450,000 noncommercial locations. To collect information on food service locations, NPD Group reviews chain directories from company headquarters, restaurant guides, industry magazines, and various business lists and conducts Internet and phone verifications. Data collection for a given establishment occurs on a rolling basis so that any one restaurant will be examined biannually. Firm-level characteristics include establishment name, exact geographic

[40]Muth and colleagues (2016) found that about 20 percent of store locations are included in InfoScan.

location, segment (i.e., quick-service versus full-service), restaurant type (e.g., hamburger, Mexican), chain membership, open date, and close date (if applicable).

Abigail Okrent, in her presentation to the panel (see Appendix B), observed that when ERS research (Levin et al., 2018) compared store counts across TDLinx, the National Establishment Time-Series (NETS) database, and InfoScan, the authors found that for the period of 2008–2012 the numbers of stores and food sales found by InfoScan were considerably lower than the numbers found by TDLinx and NETS. A comparison of these totals to totals from the 2012 Economic Census indicates that the version of InfoScan purchased by ERS covered about half of all sales at the store level.

The next two sections address, first, the strengths of commercial/proprietary data and, second, their drawbacks and disadvantages.

The Strengths of Commercial/Proprietary Data

Data originating from commercial sources provide assets for consumer food and health research and evaluation not available elsewhere. For example, retail scanner data have the advantages of providing granular food prices subject to the caveats above, geographic distribution across individual stores or markets where there is coverage, and product-level details such as brand, size/weight, type of package, health and nutrition claims (e.g., gluten-free, type of sugar added, and "good for reducing risk" of heart disease or diabetes). In the near future, such data will also likely provide information about vitamins and minerals, hormone use, and other detailed health improvement claims.[41] They also often have the advantage of providing longitudinal data and cross-time measures.[42] At the same time, as discussed below, there are weaknesses to these data.

The Food Economics Division (FED) of ERS has played a substantial role in the history of using proprietary data to estimate detailed food prices and quantities of purchases, retail sales, and consumption and purchases of food for both at-home and away-from-home eating. Data on consumer purchase transactions, retail point-of-sales, and information in food labels have been used to help answer questions about the cost of eating a healthy diet and about how the nutrient content of food products changes over time.

In collaboration with other parts of USDA, ERS has been instrumental in integrating scanner data into cost estimates and evaluations of a number of programs. Commercial data have also been applied to policy-oriented and somewhat descriptive research questions about WIC, specifically the composition of WIC-household versus non-WIC household food purchases

[41] See summary of presentation to panel by Brian Burke in Appendix B.

[42] See summary of presentation to panel by Abigail Okrent in Appendix B.

(e.g., types of products, such as breakfast cereals); use of WIC benefits by identified food items; effects of WIC program participation on food purchases; and effects on food purchases of program changes over time. Of course, identifying WIC recipients through self-reporting is less reliable than identifying them from administrative data. Projects are in place to estimate SNAP food package weights and the retail value of the average food distribution program on Indian reservations (FDPIR) using these data.[43]

Public products produced by ERS that rely on proprietary geographic data (summarized in Box 2.6) include the *Food Access Research Atlas* (FARA), *Food Environment Atlas* (FEA), and the *Quarterly Food at Home Price Database* (QFAHPD). These new geospatial databases provide new measures of food access and the food environment, such as supermarket availability, food choices, health and well-being, community characteristics, and food prices.

FARA provides a spatial overview of access to a supermarket, supercenter, or large grocery store, and thereby supports estimation of proximity to stores, both for the overall population and for subgroups of interest, such as low-income people, households without vehicles, or SNAP participants. FARA includes similar estimates refined down to the census-tract level and includes four measures of low-access census tracts, which can be overlaid with low-income tracts. This database supports the mapping of food deserts, as defined by the USDA, HHS, and the U.S. Department of Treasury as low-income census tracts with a substantial number of residents who have little access to retail outlets selling healthy and affordable foods.[44]

FEA includes more than 200 indicators, aggregated mostly at the county level, that measure both a community's ability to access healthy food and its success in doing so. Indicators include store and restaurant availability, food assistance use, food prices and taxes, local food initiatives, and residents' health and physical activity. Many of this atlas's indicators are culled from already published external data sources, but some are based on ERS data analysis.

Wilde, Llobrera, and Ver Ploeg (2014) used FARA to examine the local food retail environment in the United States. Rhone and colleagues (2017) described the changes in low-income low-food-access census tracts from 2010 to the 2015 updates to FARA. QFAHPD was used along with the ECLS-K class by Wendt and Todd (2011) to show that higher prices of sodas, 100 percent juices, starchy vegetables, and sweet snacks are associated with lower BMI, and that lower prices for dark green vegetables and

[43] See Hastings and Shapiro (2018) and Beatty and Tuttle (2015) on how SNAP benefits are spent.

[44] See https://www.ers.usda.gov/amber-waves/2011/december/data-feature-mapping-food-deserts-in-the-us.

BOX 2.6
New Products Developed by ERS since 2005

Commodity Consumption by Population Characteristics (CCPC): CCPC tracks the supply of food available for consumption in the United States and examines consumer food preferences and consumption by demographic characteristics, place where food is obtained, and food/commodity categories. See https://www.ers.usda.gov/data-products/commodity-consumption-by-population-characteristics.aspx.

Food Access Research Atlas (FARA): Uses data from TDLinx, ReCount, the FNS Store Tracking and Redemption system (STARS), and the American Community Survey to provide four estimates of proximity to stores by demographic characteristics (aggregated at the census tract level) and an indicator of low-income tracts. Users can download census tract data. See https://www.ers.usda.gov/data-products/food-access-research-atlas.

Food Consumption and Nutrient Intake Database by Population Characteristics: Offers data tables showing food consumption and food density as well as average daily intake of nutrients by food source and demographic characteristics. See https://www.ers.usda.gov/data-products/food-consumption-and-nutrient-intakes.

Food Environment Atlas (FEA): Includes more than 200 indicators of a community's ability to access healthy food and its success in doing so, covering characteristics such as store and restaurant availability, food assistance use, food prices and taxes, local foods initiatives, and health and physical activity. Data are at the county level for most indicators. Many indicators are from already published external data sources. Users can download the data. See https://www.ers.usda.gov/foodatlas.

Price Spreads from Farm to Consumer: Compares prices paid by consumers for food (based on Homescan and the BLS Consumer Expenditure Survey) with prices received by farmers for corresponding commodities. See https://www.ers.usda.gov/data-products/price-spreads-from-farm-to-consumer.

Quarterly Food at Home Price Database (QFAHPD): Provides prices for more than 50 food groups based on scanner data for 26 metropolitan markets and 9 nonmetropolitan markets. Users can download the data. See https://www.ers.usda.gov/data-products/quarterly-food-at-home-price-database.aspx. Provides access to state-level SNAP eligibility rules and administrative policies as well as distribution schedules. See https://www.ers.usda.gov/data-products/snap-policy-data-sets.

Retail Fruit and Vegetable Prices: Provides estimates for average costs of fruits and vegetables using 2013 and 2016 proprietary InfoScan data. See https://www.ers.usda.gov/data-products/fruit-and-vegetable-prices/documentation.

SNAP Policy Database: Provides access to state-level SNAP eligibility rules and administrative policies as well as distribution schedules. See https://www.ers.usda.gov/data-products/snap-policy-data-sets.

low-fat milk are also associated with reduced BMI; by Todd and colleagues (2011) to describe geographic differences in the prices of healthy foods; by Gregory and Coleman-Jensen (2013) to show that food insecurity was higher in areas with higher food prices; and with NHIS by Bronchetti and colleagues (2019) to show that lower SNAP purchasing power (because of higher prices) leads to a lower utilization of preventative care among children and more days of school missed due to illness.

The databases summarized in Box 2.6 also support enhancing sample designs and adding new variables to survey data. ERS added important additional value by extensively evaluating coverage—both geographically and across other dimensions—through comparisons of these data with Census data on sales in the retail trade and other sources. Comparisons that have been made with total sales from the Census of Retail Trade and other sources suggest that total spending is under-reported in scanner data.[45] While some of these databases span nearly the whole country, others are limited in their geographic coverage. For example, Nielsen's Homescan predominately covers large markets.[46]

The application of commercial data to the study of food, nutrition, and health topics is now commonplace. Mary Muth, in a presentation to the panel,[47] identified more than 150 peer-reviewed publications using some form of scanner and/or label data for food policy research topics. Because no other comparable data source provides the same level of granularity, detail, and frequency, which is needed for many types of food policy analyses, scanner data will continue to be important in a range of research policy areas. Specifically, scanner data can be used

- to analyze the effects of federal regulations on the healthiness of food acquired (e.g., new Nutrition Facts Labels, revised serving sizes, and the banning of partially hydrogenated oils [trans fatty acids] as an ingredient);
- as inputs in analyses of new labeling regulations assessing the benefits of changing consumption and the costs (estimated elsewhere) of implementing these changes;
- to analyze the effects of local regulations, such as taxes on sugar-sweetened beverages, on consumption and to evaluate the incidence of such policies;

[45] Mary Muth presentation to the panel; see Appendix C.

[46] For excerpts from an ERS report, see http://qed.econ.queensu.ca/jae/2007-v22.7/hausman-leibtag/Homescan-data.

[47] See Appendix C for a summary of this presentation.

- to analyze, in a descriptive manner, the effects of voluntary industry initiatives, such as the Healthy Convenience Store Initiative;[48]
- to analyze impacts of food contamination outbreaks on sales; and
- to calculate price indices for a broad range of research studies, to the extent that they incorporate individual prices as well as commodities.

Drawbacks and Challenges in Using Commercial/Proprietary Data

While commercial data will certainly play a growing role in food research, measurement, and assessment, there are considerable hurdles to their use that will need to be overcome before such data can be used as the "gold standard" and in longitudinal assessments. These hurdles include access issues, bias in coverage and representation, perpetually dynamic algorithms, lack of documentation and transparency, fake data and bots, limited scope of organic data sources, and privacy concerns. Each is discussed next, in turn.

Access Issues

One of the most difficult aspects of using commercial or nonfederal administrative data is the challenge of accessing data sources (see National Academies of Sciences, Engineering and Medicine, 2017a). The potential roadblocks are many: propriety information concerning how a dataset was created and unwillingness to share or sell the details, limiting conditions of privacy, restrictions that limit use by some public universities (discussed in Chapter 4), lack of a central data repository, and disparate versions of seemingly similar data (such as refrigerator sensor data that vary across makes and models).

Among the easiest types of data to access are nonfederal administrative data from open data sources; commoditized data; and certain types of social media data (in particular, Twitter). Next easiest to access are data that can be obtained from a single proprietor, although these often require considerable negotiation, contract use restrictions, and time. This latter category includes administrative records from states or organizations; commercial transactions and e-commerce; and health or medical records. Among the most difficult data to access consistently are data derived from social media (such as Facebook or Instagram), web logs, and the so-called Internet of things.

---

[48]See https://midsouthgreenprint.org/greenprint-20152040/subplanning-projects/healthy-convenience-store-initiative.

Coverage and Representation Bias

For any research to produce valid and reliable conclusions, it is critical that the data and assessments be representative of the populations or subpopulations of interest and that the degree of representativeness be known or noted. For this reason, ERS has conducted or commissioned research to better understand the characteristics of commercial data sources. In some commercial databases there are gaps in coverage. For instance, Leibtag and Kauffman (2003) and Lusk and Brooks (2011) have documented underrepresentation of lower-income consumers in the Nielsen panel. At the retail level, some data exclude smaller independent stores or private-label products, which make up nearly 18 percent of all food purchases (Cuffey and Beatty, 2019). In terms of scanner data, there can be difficulties in identifying critical groups of interest, such as low-income households, working parents, WIC recipients, or even those who are WIC eligible but not participating in the program (Jensen, 2018).

The method or mode by which data are collected can also be a concern, leading to underrepresentation. For instance, for the populations that ERS wants to follow, it remains an open question whether online data collection methods are a viable option, for example because of unfamiliarity with the use of computers and online methods. Another issue may be that individuals are afraid of having their information in a database and/or fear that may lead to some form of reprisal (such as deportation). Nonresponse or lack of participation by program participants can lead to underrepresentation in the statistics produced.

Using a comparison of sales from the Economic Census to the IRI/Nielson consumer panel data, Muth[49] showed that the consumer panel underrepresents sales, particularly for random-weight products such as fresh fruits and vegetables. There are also challenges with using a dataset like the consumer network panel, whose proprietors themselves use "projection factors" or weights derived from proprietary sources or constructed in a proprietary fashion to make the data comparable to national totals for demographics. If these factors or weights are suppressed when the data are made available for use, this is limiting. Comparisons of retail proprietary data and Nielsen Homescan data have also been reported to show discrepancies, as found by Einav, Leibtag, and Nevo (2010), who propose corrections for researchers using Nielsen Homescan data.

Perpetual Dynamic Algorithm

While nonsurvey/nonadministrative data can often provide useful analyses, it is important to remember that many of these data are derived

[49]See summary of Muth's presentation to the panel in Appendix C.

from information required to run a system or carry out a process. Regular changes in the platform mechanics and algorithms used to drive these systems reflect the reality that these systems are in place for a business or platform purpose, not for the end goal of generating high-quality research data.

The problem this presents is that changes in data resulting from engineering or programming modifications are often (i) unknown to the researchers and (ii) impossible to disentangle from actual changes in human behaviors, attitudes, or transactions (Lazer et al., 2014). There is a similar issue when proprietary data products change or offer different versions over time.[50] There can be a loss of—or significant change in—a data source or a production system, which then leads to different conclusions being drawn.[51] One practical example involves the difficulty in making cross-time comparisons when manufacturers assign a new barcode to an existing product (which may be done when a product undergoes a substantial change of some sort). This can make it difficult to separate new products on the market from older ones that have a new label.[52]

Lack of Documentation and Transparency of Method

Organic data often lack the traditional types of documentation researchers are used to having or may have no documentation at all. This applies not only to the potential fields of data but also, perhaps more importantly, to the ability to trace the origins of the data or changes made to the data at various points before reaching the researcher. This can fundamentally undermine the ability to fully understand what the data actually represent, both conceptually and population-wise, and also limits assessments of data quality.

Fake Data/Bots

The problems caused by bots and fake accounts are ubiquitous within the social media and Internet space. They cause contamination by generating false information either automatically by machine or through use of a cadre of people and are generally designed to push a particular perspective or piece of information. This is particularly problematic in the realm of social media, where platforms are generally open and have fairly low thresholds for entry, leaving themselves vulnerable (Japec et al., 2015). Researchers interested in leveraging social media or scraping websites to gain greater

---

[50]See Appendix C for a summary of the presentation by Alessandro Bonanno.
[51]See Appendix C for a summary of the presentation by John Eltinge.
[52]See Appendix C for a summary of the presentation by Mary Muth.

understanding of food-relevant issues need to take such approaches with care. Although there are commercial packages that claim to help identify fake accounts and bot-generated data, the results of such efforts often conflict across various software packages, thereby rendering such services unreliable for assessing data quality.

Limited Scope of Organic Data Sources

While organic data can often provide very granular and timely data, the information they offer is often of limited scope, being rich in just a small set of variables. Researchers typically have much broader needs, wanting to understand a range of concepts, interactions, and often motivations. The need to understand the "why" behind attitudes and behaviors is still quite germane, but often it is not knowable from organic data alone. For example, scanner data tend not to include whole classes of goods, such as non-UPC products like fresh fruit and vegetables (Jensen, 2018), so it is difficult to assess attitudinal and behavioral changes related to the selection of these mostly healthy alternatives. To remedy this, such data are often best utilized in combination with richer data from surveys or more complete administrative records.

Privacy Concerns

As with nearly all forms of data related to individuals, there is concern about the privacy of the individuals whose data are used. This is a particularly complex issue when commercial and other forms of organic data are used. In those instances, the individuals are rarely (if ever) notified about the potential uses of their data—and even when they are informed, such as through a use agreement, they rarely understand the ultimate implications of potentially sharing their data with others. This is also an area where many laws and regulations have not kept pace with the technology and forms of data generated from these systems and devices. Researchers are therefore urged to approach such usage with caution and take what steps they can to protect the privacy of those whose data are being used.

2.4. NUTRIENT/FOOD COMPOSITION DATABASES

ARS, in collaboration with ERS, FNS, USDA's Center for Nutrition Policy and Promotion, NCHS, the National Cancer Institute, and others, develops and maintains nutrient/food composition databases or "crosswalk" databases (tables or databases that show the relationship between variables in other tables or databases). Selected food composition databases are listed in Box 2.7. For example, the Food and Nutrient Database for

BOX 2.7
Selected USDA Food Composition Databases

Branded Food Products Database (BFPDB): Result of a public-private partnership to provide nutrient composition of branded foods and private label data provided by the food industry. Covers 229,064 branded products from 238 food categories.

Food and Nutrient Database for Dietary Studies (FNDDS): FNDDS identifies the nutrient profiles for 8,000 foods and beverages reported on NHANES. ARS is supposed to release FNDDS every 2 years in concert with the 2-year releases of NHANES.

Food Intakes Converted to Retail Commodities database (FICRCD): FICRCD translates the foods in FNDDS into 65 food commodities at the retail level, as defined by ERS. There are two versions of the database, one based on The Continuing Survey of Food Intake by Individuals (CSFII) 1994–1996 and 1998; NHANES 1999–2000; and What We Eat in America (WWEIA)/NHANES 2001–2002, the other based on the NHANES 2003–2008.

Food Patterns Equivalent Database (FPED): FPED translates foods and beverages in FNDDS into the 37 USDA food pattern groups that have been defined by CNPP based on the dietary guidelines for Americans. Databases available for 2005–2006, 2007–2008, 2009–2010, 2011–2012, 2013–2014, 2015–2016. Updates are typically released with the new FNDDS.

National Nutrient Database for Standard Reference Legacy Release (NNDSR): Includes information on nutrient availability (more than 66 nutrients) for more than 7,000 foods and foods groups. Includes amounts of nutrients (water, protein, fats by type, sugars by type, vitamins, minerals, etc.) per 100 grams of a food or food group.

Dietary Studies (FNDDS) identifies the nutrient profiles for 8,000 foods and beverages reported on NHANES. The Food Intakes Converted to Retail Commodities Database (FICRCD) crosswalks the foods and beverages on FNDDS into 65 food commodities (foods directly related to agriculture). These databases are or will be available in USDA's FoodData Central.[53] They are used to add new variables to already collected survey data.

Andrea Carlson, in her presentation to the panel (see summary in Appendix A), described the collaborative project with USDA's Center for Nutrition Policy and Promotion and Agricultural Statistics Service (ARS) to integrate ARS food composition databases with IRI scanner data to support creation of prices for foods consumed (as collected in NHANES) (Carlson

[53]Link to FoodData Central: see https://fdc.nal.usda.gov/index.html. Link to Food Surveys Research Group, ARS: see https://www.ars.usda.gov/northeast-area/beltsville-md-bhnrc/beltsville-human-nutrition-research-center/food-surveys-research-group/docs/fndds-download-databases.

et al., 2019). One purpose was to evaluate the prices and nutritional composition of foods associated with the *Dietary Guidelines for Americans*, especially MyPlate recommendations. The project created the purchase-to-plate crosswalk via the Food Purchase and Acquisition Groups, now called ERS Food Purchase Groups (EFPG), which assign IRI UPC codes to USDA-related food groups based on ingredients, nutritional content, convenience to consumer, and store aisle. An early version of this database and the Nielsen scanner data were used to prepare the QFAHPD to compute quarterly estimates of the prices of 52 food categories. These categories include three categories of fruit—fresh or frozen fruit, canned fruit, and fruit juices—and nine categories of vegetables for 35 regional market groups at several points in time. ERS plans to expand scanner data applications. For example, EFPGs could be included in future iterations of FoodAPS for purposes of food environment studies.

The project also created a price tool for the FNDDS, which estimates prices for the individual foods in FNDDS using scanner data. This tool supports analysis of the relationship between food prices and nutritional content. FNDDS and similar tools have been used to augment publicly available data from existing surveys.

The USDA Branded Food Products Database (BFPDB) was described by Alison Krester and Kyle McKillop at the panel's second workshop (see Appendix B). The goal of the project is to enhance public health and the sharing of open data by complementing the ARS National Nutrient Database with information on the nutrient composition of branded foods and private label data provided by the food industry.[54] The BFPDB covers 229,064 branded products from 238 food categories. Linking the BFPDB to specific years of NHANES surveys, if possible, could more accurately assess dietary intake within the United States. Having a historical record of branded and private-label foods enables comparisons of current and past consumption.

In her presentation to the panel (see Appendix B), Susan Krebs-Smith of the National Cancer Institute illustrated the value added by these crosswalk databases by explaining their application in estimating HEI scores. The HEI is designed to measure conformance of the diets of the U.S. population with the *Dietary Guidelines for Americans*, which is published every 5 years and which USDA is a partner in creating. The index can be computed for any given basket of food items, whether that is foods consumed, foods purchased, or food commodities.

The HEI is made up of 13 food group components: total fruits, whole fruits, total vegetables, greens and beans, whole grains, dairy, total protein foods, seafood and plant proteins, fatty acids, refined grains, sodium, added sugars, and saturated fats. Weights for constructing the index were derived

---

[54]See https://data.nal.usda.gov/dataset/usda-branded-food-products-database.

from the *Dietary Guidelines for Americans*. To generate a total HEI score for a person or group, information on the quantities of all food groups consumed is needed. The index's aim is to determine the balance among food groups, including the nine food groups to encourage, such as fruits and vegetables, and the four to reduce, such as discretionary fats and added sugars. A person (group) can improve their HEI score by consuming more of the foods to encourage (these enter the HEI with a positive weight) and by decreasing consumption of the foods to discourage (these add to the HEI if consumed in moderation).

One advantage of the HEI is that scores can be constructed at different levels in the food supply chain, from the agricultural commodities produced by farmers to the food based on those commodities consumed by ultimate consumers and anything in between. In order to examine the HEI at different levels of the food chain, the foods or commodities at that level need to be identified and classified into the 13 categories of the HEI. In his presentation to the panel, Biing-Hwan Lin described translating the data from the ERS Food Availability (per capita) Data System (FADS) to assess the nutritional value of agricultural products produced by farmers and delivered for consumption (see Appendix B). FADS includes data on commodity flows from producer to end user to produce national estimates of the amounts of commodities that are available for consumption by end-users through all channels. It is a proxy for consumption.[55] Lin noted that agricultural producers are interested in knowing who consumes their commodities, where they are consumed, and how they are served. Whereas food consumption surveys cover store-bought foods, including fresh produce and meats but also boxed and prepared foods (e.g., cake mix and apple pie), they do not cover the constituent commodities (e.g., apples, wheat, butter, sugar) of those prepared and boxed foods. FADS measures 200 food commodity supplies through the supply chain from the farmer to domestic consumption. The project described by Lin combined food consumption data from NHANES for 2007–2010 with the Food Intakes Converted to Retail Commodities Database and Food Patterns Equivalent Database to estimate food consumption by food groups as specified in the 2010 *Dietary Guidelines for Americans*. ERS has published statistics covering the years 1994 through 2008 in *Commodity Consumption by Population Characteristics*,[56] using FADS and NHANES data to generate information about the roles of

[55]The ERS loss-adjusted food availability (LAFA) data are derived from the FADS data by subtracting out estimates of food spoilage, plate waste, and other losses to more closely approximate consumption. LAFA is called a preliminary series by ERS because the loss estimates could be improved.

[56]See https://www.ers.usda.gov/data-products/commodity-consumption-by-population-characteristics/documentation.

agricultural commodities versus food and food policy effects on producers and consumers for various demographic characteristics.

For some levels of the food chain, the linkage between foods (whether grown, sold, or consumed) and nutrients or the HEI can be made using one or more of the nutrition databases. For example, constructing the HEI for FADS requires using data from NNDSR, FICRCD, and the U.S. Salt Institute. Constructing the HEI for food consumption data from NHANES requires using data from the FPED and the FNDDS. Crosswalk databases are still needed for food processing and for the community food environment. For example, packaged brownie mix and macaroni and cheese in a box need to be translated into food-pattern equivalents along with nutrient data.

With the appropriate crosswalks, the HEI can be used to evaluate the "diet quality" associated with grocery store purchases, with grocery store circulars, with the places where food is obtained (e.g., different kinds of restaurants or fast food outlets), with schools, with food pantries, and so on. In addition to being used for surveillance and monitoring, the HEI could be used to analyze the relationships between diet patterns and health outcomes. One example of the latter analysis is that of Mancino and colleagues (2018), who use the HEI to assess the quality of food acquired. Fang and colleagues (2019) also use FoodAPS to describe the healthfulness of food acquired by WIC recipients (although they call it the Health Purchasing Index), and Frisvold and Price (2019) use the HEI to characterize the healthfulness of school meals offered by the bulk of schools.

3

Data and Knowledge Gaps

The Consumer Food Data System (CFDS), produced by the Food and Economics Division of the Economic Research Service (ERS), can provide data, fill information holes, and facilitate science in three areas. First, as a statistical agency, ERS can use the CFDS to carry out a series of monitoring tasks that allow the public, policy makers, and researchers to track outcomes across time. Second, CFDS can be used to assess the quality and coverage properties of various types of data, including data collected by other agencies. Assessing the quality of data used within ERS's Food Economics Division, in the statistical agencies more broadly, and by outside researchers in turn improves the quality of research.

The third area where the CFDS can contribute is in the creation of data and the carrying out of research by ERS and other USDA staff as well as outside researchers. Specifically, the CFDS can enable statistical approaches in the study of both descriptive and causal questions, particularly as they pertain to programs designed to improve the well-being of persons across the United States. Descriptive evidence establishes facts and terms of debates and provides hypotheses for further research. Causal designs provide evidence of the outcomes made possible by USDA programs. Of particular value is the way the CFDS can strengthen researchers' ability to conduct evaluations of both current food assistance programs and potential future interventions.

In this chapter, each of these three functional areas is described. While, Chapter 4 explicitly presents strategies for improving the CFDS, this chapter describes in more general terms data areas warranting further attention by ERS and the statistical system more broadly.

3.1. MONITORING NEEDS

Producing data that allow the monitoring of food and nutrition outcomes, together with related health outcomes, and using these and other data to create snapshots of the population's nutritional and other food-related health, are key components of the CFDS. These snapshots also help stakeholders to understand trends in these areas over time. In addition, when monitoring data are available at more granular levels, state and local information—such as that complied for the Food Access Atlas, discussed in Chapter 2—can be created.

Food Security

The first subject area for which the CFDS provides crucial data related to monitoring population outcomes, particularly through the December Current Population Survey (DCPS), is the measurement of food security. The DCPS data collection instrument enables annual snapshots of food security by state and by various demographic and economic measures over a long time period, but there are holes in its existing measurement of food security. One drawback is that the DCPS is only conducted during 1 month of the year, December. That choice does have the advantage of providing consistent estimates across years, helping to mitigate the wide oscillations that occur in the Current Population Survey (CPS) depending on which month is used to measure food insecurity. But in light of these oscillations, in order to monitor seasonal patterns, it would be extremely useful to collect the Core Food Security Module during other months of the DCPS, at least occasionally. A particularly important gap is our understanding of the experiences of households with children during the summer months, when school meal programs are not available.

Additional important data are provided by including various measures of food security on a range of other surveys beyond the DCPS. One of the most useful is the National Health and Nutrition Examination Survey (NHANES), which also generates objective measures of health (participating individuals have their health measured objectively by professionals). This allows researchers to see how food security varies with objective and subjective measures of health. This feature of the survey is important, given that some individuals might not know about health conditions that they have if they do not see a medical professional frequently. However, NHANES uses only small samples, limiting the ability of researchers to correlate these health measures with food security to help understand its ramifications. Moreover, in part due to these small sample sizes, NHANES is only nationally representative in demographic terms and lacks the detailed geographic information needed to measure at the state and substate level. In practice, data are collected for a limited number of counties each year.

This lack of state-level representativeness means that different years of NHANES may include people from entirely different state and local policy settings, complicating standard two-way fixed-effects model designs,[1] which require repeated measures from many of the same locations over time. NHANES surveys persons from a small number of counties each year, so it would not allow for such fine granularity unless its sample sizes were increased. These small samples across locations limit the array of analyses. National Center for Health Statistics (NCHS) is responsible for NHANES and deciding sample sizes and questions; however, in the past, ERS has sponsored modules that expanded samples.

Similarly, there are disadvantages, especially for child-focus analyses and replicability with other datasets, to having the National Health Interview Survey (NHIS) not include all 18 questions but only the 10 food security items asked of adult respondents in the NHIS Food Security Module at the annual level (rather than 30 day). Were the NHIS instead to have 18 rather than 10 items, it would greatly enhance the extensive health information collected in the NHIS. It would also allow for research on the effects of long-term health problems and disability on food insecurity or the effects of food insecurity on more short-term health outcomes be advanced.

The Panel Survey of Income Dynamics (PSID) also monitors food security. The only nationally representative longitudinal dataset that uses the full 18-question food security instrument, it includes detailed measures of individuals' income, employment, health, wealth, consumption, food expenditures, and family structure in a panel fashion. While the CPS data allow for longitudinal analysis of repeated cross-sections, the PSID measures the same people over time, allowing for more precise measure of changes in outcomes than repeated cross-sections (e.g., Duncan and Kalton, 1987). If the PSID discontinued questions about food insecurity, it would leave gaps in the data sources used for tracking it.

[1]Such regression models are used for estimating causal effects from panel data. The simplest case of such a two-way fixed-effects model compares outcomes for two populations and two time periods. In this simplest model (also known as differences in differences), the goal is to understand the effects of a policy change or treatment that takes please in the second time period for one of the groups (the treated group). The simplest approach would be to take the difference in the treated group before and after the policy change (a difference). But the concern with doing only that is that other shocks occurring at the same time as the policy change would confound this simple difference. If the control group also faces the same shocks, however, then the change in the control group serves as a counterfactual for what would have happened in the treated group in the absence of the policy change, and the resulting difference in difference provides a causal estimate of the effects of the policy. This can be generalized to a setting with many periods and groups, where the group-fixed effects control for time-invariant factors in each group and the time-fixed effects control for period-specific shocks that all the groups face, yielding the terminology "two-way fixed effects" models.

Program Rules about Food Assistance and Other USDA Activities

Another missing link in the monitoring area is the absence of a comprehensive set of measures of rules affecting participants, firms, and nonprofit providers, such as schools and clinics, in the food assistance network in the United States, including those that participate in the Special Supplemental Nutrition Program for Women, Infants, and Children (WIC). ERS has collected data on both eligibility policy and disbursement policy for the Supplemental Nutrition Assistance Program (SNAP), which have led to a host of papers studying the effects of these policies on health, education, food security, and economic outcomes. But these rules are not always updated annually, and the data only cover SNAP to date and leave out the other important child nutrition programs. An important missing link is an accounting of the state- and county-level choices about rules for the participation of individuals in these other programs, such as WIC, the school meal programs, the Child and Adult Care Food Program (CACFP), summer feeding programs, and other USDA programs at the relevant geographic and temporal level for modelling eligibility. This would enable researchers within and outside of USDA to measure how changes in rules affect use of programs; it would also enable them to model disaggregated measures of program eligibility. ERS is also limited in its ability to go to the state, county, and local entities administering these programs due to limits on burden, although the USDA Food and Nutrition Service (FNS) knows more about these programs in many cases. It would also help research to be able to document where local, state, or federal eligibility decisions are made, for example by listing the locations of SNAP offices.

In addition, some of these food assistance programs affect a set of nonprofit organizations that administer the programs, such as schools (school meals programs), CACFP facilities, and WIC clinics. It is also important to understand how these rules affect the choices made by these nonprofits. One example would be the Community Eligibility Program (CEP), which enables schools with sufficiently high levels of students eligible for free and reduced-price meals to choose to offer free meals to all students with a federal subsidy. As part of this program, states are required to make the lists of schools that qualify for this new option publicly available. Currently, these lists of CEP-eligible schools are available from the nonprofit Food Research and Action Center,[2] having them collected by and made available through ERS would be a more natural choice. Another example of the kind of data that it would seem natural for FED to collect is the *timing and choices for meal pattern requirements* for CACFP or school meals to be reimbursed for meals/snacks provided, disaggregated by detailed geography and time.

---

[2] See https://www.frac.org/cep-map/cep-map.html.

To know how these nutrition policies affect food choices, one must have information about where and when they apply, including when they are enacted and actually implemented.

Food assistance programs, mainly SNAP and WIC, also affect businesses such as convenience stores, grocery stores, and larger chains. Firms choose to participate in these programs by providing food in return for payments from customers using Electronic Benefits Transfer (EBT) card payments or, in the case of WIC, paper vouchers, for which the firms are then reimbursed. Here, there is a wide set of questions that would be useful to address. These questions range from knowing whether the state requires WIC-authorized stores to participate in SNAP, to what options the state has selected for the WIC cash-value vouchers for fruits and vegetables, to when the state implemented other rules such as for EBT use and what form EBT takes for SNAP and WIC. Information about these rules, and how states interpret the rules, helps researchers understand varying eligibility status across states as well as the administrative burden of program participation (for firms, nonprofits, and potential participants). Having an accurate accounting of the firm rules is also important for studying how stores choose to participate in or leave specific programs. In addition, knowing which firms are potentially eligible to participate allows researchers to see where there are gaps in access to consumers and how these gaps may affect the prices faced by participating individuals. Finally, as EBT is implemented for WIC, states have more information about what individuals purchase using WIC vouchers, and it should already be possible to see what individuals purchase with SNAP. This could fill gaps in our knowledge of what food assistance programs facilitate.

Program Participation and Eligibility, and Locations Where Eligibility Is Determined

To understand program use, it is important to have geographic and time measures with fine detail on program participation and eligibility. USDA provides researchers, policy makers, and the public with snapshots of outcomes such as participation among individuals eligible for SNAP, available at the state level and nationally by group. Data on participation in WIC (program characteristics data) and demographic and state measures of take-up for WIC (reports) are also available. Yet more fine-grained counts of participation refined by demographic and geographic detail and, if possible, by eligibility would add value by pinpointing where targeting has been useful and where it is failing. Of course, measuring eligibility among nonparticipants is challenging. Some of the components that would enable this to be done for participation already exist but are not easily accessible or are only available by restricted geographic aggregations (e.g., the WIC

Participant and Program Characteristics). Other measures of eligibility are produced at the state level by contractors for FNS.

It is important to know where the various programs are available. This would include having access to a list of stores that historically have participated in WIC or SNAP without requiring a Freedom of Information Act (FOIA) request. It would also include having access to information about stores that have been sanctioned from the program as well as lists of schools participating in the School Breakfast and National School Lunch programs, of child and adult care facilities that use CACFP, and of locations participating in the summer feeding program. Some of these lists are currently available but only as snapshots, whereas causal research requires having historical data too. These measures of access to free and reduced-price food allow researchers and stakeholders to see where benefits are available and how that geography compares to where eligible participants and nonparticipants live. Access to data on stores on and off the programs allows researchers to study how firms participate and also how sanctions affect firms and participants.

In addition, a list of charitable food agencies would be useful for the purpose of understanding the larger food environment. The food banks under the Feeding America network (and the agencies under those food banks) constitute the overwhelming majority of charitable food assistance in the United States. Feeding America has information on these food banks and their locations, as well as about their hours of service, number of people served, and so on. A data-sharing partnership with this network would therefore help achieve this data collection objective.

It is also important to know where the agents who assess eligibility for food assistance programs are located. In the case of schools, this is included in one of the above lists. But SNAP eligibility is assessed at county SNAP offices, and WIC eligibility is assessed at WIC clinics. These data should also be aggregated to allow research monitoring access and also on how access affects use of programs and ultimately, participant outcomes. Combined with this information, knowing where eligible and participating people are located would also be useful. Ideally, information would be detailed enough to ascertain who is eligible for SNAP, WIC, and other programs at a fine geographic level, such as by county, as well as who is participating in these programs and how this is affected by the food and program eligibility determination environment.

Finally, how these programs interact with one another is often not well understood. For example, joint participation by individuals and households in SNAP and some other non-USDA program can be assessed using quality control data, and similar joint participation in WIC and some other programs can be viewed in the WIC PC data. However, outside of survey data, which struggle to count each program accurately, and these eligibility determination administrative data, joint participation is hard to measure.

Measuring it better would allow improved research on a number of policy issues ranging from eligibility determinations to program effects on child outcomes and the inability to do so represents a current gap.

A gap in the data infrastructure on program participation is the lack of guidance for compiling a list of and then updating policies over time. Ideally, there would be a standardized scheme for including policies, a method for geocoding all locations, and a method for managing timestamps and providing version control. Sound data management would improve efficient processing and dissemination for researchers and policy makers.

The Food Environment

Another valuable innovation from USDA is the *Food Access Research Atlas,* one of the agency's most widely used collections of data provided to the public.[3] This atlas reports at two points in time where the prevalence of retail food outlets is available at the census tract level. Having repeated cross-sectional measures of the types of food available by store is important, as it allows researchers to study access.

Currently, data from IRI and Nielsen do a good job of obtaining this information. The challenge in accessing this data, however, is three-fold. First, purchasing the data from IRI or Nielsen can be prohibitively expensive for many researchers, especially those at less wealthy institutions, limiting the number of researchers with access and, in turn, the set of questions that can be posed. Second, while the sampling frame for the IRI and Nielsen data does include some smaller stores, these data are not released to outside researchers because they are highly proprietary.[4] Even though overall coverage may be good, especially for non-low-income households, some stores, especially those that may disproportionately be located in low-income neighborhoods, may be overlooked. Perhaps methods could be used to incentivize IRI and Nielsen to include these stores in their sampling frames. The most valuable way to do that might be to lower the sales volume needed to be included in the sample, an approach that would not necessarily require including specific stores. Another part of the problem is that stores enter and exit the sample, and smaller stores are most likely to experience this. Greater retention of small stores in the sample would therefore be helpful. A third issue is that IRI requires researchers to sign indemnity clauses to use its data, when linked to FoodAPS, and Nielsen has

[3] For a detailed description of the *Atlas*, see Chapter 2 and a summary of the presentation to the panel by Michele Ver Ploeg in Appendix A.

[4] In general, coverage in rural areas is limited. For example, for counties with 20,000 or fewer residents, Nielsen uses an average of the surrounding counties. This is a "rural issue" insofar as these counties have fewer stores, but it is not, strictly speaking, due to the sampling methods used by Nielsen.

similar requirements for TDLinx. Most state universities will not sign such clauses as they violate state law, restricting who can work on these topics.

Measures such as those indicating the presence of certain types of stores by detailed geography also might serve as indicators of the set of firms "at risk" for participating in SNAP or WIC.[5] It is also important that researchers, policy makers, and other stakeholders can identify where stores and other entities that participate in the program are geographically located so that the information can be combined with data about the location and stores at risk of participating (see above point). Combined data would allow researchers to investigate whether there are places where food programs are not present but where people and stores are. It would also let researchers study how the food environment is affected when stores are temporarily or permanently kicked off WIC or SNAP.

Similarly, data such as which schools are participating in universal meals or school breakfasts also should be available and could conceivably be added to such data dissemination vehicles as the National Center for Education Statistics Common Core database or the Food Security Supplement of the Current Population Survey. Going forward, the food environment is sure to change as families increasingly use delivery services such as Amazon, Grub Hub, or Blue Apron. It is also useful to know where various providers of free food (pantries) are located as well as where restaurants (by level of healthfulness) are available at fine geography in order to study consumer choices.

Another component of the food environment is the broader set of expenditures facing vulnerable households. Consider the problem of food insecurity. Over one-half of poor households are food secure, while approximately 15 percent of nonpoor households are food insecure. This is due to many factors that are often observed in datasets, but the influence of other expenditures is often not observed on the same datasets that record food insecurity. Of particular note might be the expenditures households make on housing, which vary dramatically across the United States. Another factor that varies is transportation costs. Information on both of these could be included in the geographic landscape dataset mentioned above.

Consumption

It is also important to understand how restaurants, stores, and the rest of the food environment affect consumer demand. This includes understanding demand for product attributes, such as whether foods are locally

[5]Given that nearly all stores receive SNAP, this is more of a WIC issue than a SNAP issue. Although, it is true that a small share of stores are removed from each program when they violate rules.

produced, natural, or organic. Other examples of relevant questions include these: How do consumers value and use side-of-the-package information, such as nutrition facts? How do they use front-of-the-package health claims (e.g., "heart healthy")? How do they value production characteristics, such as whether foods are organic or hormone-free? And, How do they value other characteristics (e.g., "natural")? Understanding these questions requires data about the characteristics or attributes of food—such as that which has been collected in IRI data and, prior to that, in the Gladstone data—as well as the ingredients. This is discussed further in Chapter 4. This would also encompass questions such as understanding demand for novel products, such as plant-based meat alternatives, and how this affects the food system.

Prices

Food choices are affected by availability, income, and the characteristics of the food environment—each discussed above. Another element affecting food choice is, of course, pricing. The Bureau of Labor Statistics (BLS) collects excellent data on prices for urban areas but has limited coverage of rural areas. Knowing the prices for foods at refined geographic levels is important for understanding the value of food assistance benefits and for monitoring the performance of programs that administer therm. For example, breaking down purchased foods into "healthful" and "unhealthful" categories can be useful.

For 34 geographic regions, price indices (levels and changes) were provided by USDA's Quarterly Food at Home Data. However, these data undoubtedly miss within-market variation in prices; moreover, this information has not been updated since 2012 and lacks detail about variety concerning what food types appear within each category. Datasets derived from scanners report weekly prices, but some level of detail is suppressed for many stores or only averages are provided. So, while these scanner data are far more disaggregated than most of the data obtainable from existing government sources, and while they represent the average shopping experience, they do not necessarily contain individual variation in prices paid. Data on individual prices paid at specific stores, net of taxes and other features like coupons, would let researchers know where food prices are high, allow them to measure the pass-through of factors affecting prices to consumers, and let them measure the incidence of the food assistance programs. Additionally, when collecting prices and building price indices, it is important that particular attention be paid to items that will improve the reference diets.

There is one example of price data that are already available that may be useful for program monitoring. As part of Feeding America's Map the

Meal Gap,[6] which maps food insecurity rates by county and congressional district for each state, Nielsen data are used by USDA to compile the price of the Thrifty Food Plan for all counties in the United States.[7] The Thrifty Food Plan is designed by USDA to specify foods and amounts of foods that provide adequate nutrition in a way that provides the basis for determining the monetary value of SNAP benefits.[8] While data on the Thrifty Food Plan do not provide the level of disaggregation needed for some analyses, they can be employed in other cases, such as SNAP analyses. The value of these data would be even greater if they could be linked to the December CPS (or NHANES or NHIS) within the Research Data System. One additional benefit of working with Nielsen to ensure that more stores are covered (in the manner described above) is the potential to improve measurements of the Thrifty Food Plan.

Time Costs

Food choices are also affected by time costs (both distance and travel time to food acquisition venues) and the time it takes to prepare food. Time cost is particularly important given that food assistance program benefits are in-kind and, in the case of SNAP, they can only include food items that are not already prepared. BLS's American Time Use Survey (ATUS) provides a useful snapshot of time use, and the eating and health module to ATUS also captures eating when it is a secondary activity (e.g., while watching TV) but includes no other useful features. Secondary eating (eating while doing other activities) is understudied in time use data.

FoodAPS documented that the usual store for a family's food purchases is only 3.8 miles away from their home and that the vast bulk of individuals use a car to shop even when they do not own one (Ver Ploeg et al., 2015). Yet little is known about the time costs of travel to stores, which includes both driving time and waiting time. The tradeoffs between time and money in food acquisition would be useful to know. In the same way, it is also hard to model the administrative burden of programs on recipients, firms, or lower levels of government or nonprofits administering programs without knowing the administrative time costs of their participation.

---

[6] See https://map.feedingamerica.org.

[7] Among small counties, some do not have any stores, and even among those that do none of the stores is included in the Nielsen dataset, so all counties with fewer than 20,000 residents are represented by a weighted average of the county itself combined with its surrounding counties.

[8] See https://www.fns.usda.gov/cnpp/usda-food-plans-cost-food-reports.

Food-Related Health Measurement

Finally, there are various other food-related health measures beyond food insecurity that are crucial for modeling the effects of programs, the food environment, and prices on food choice, consumption, and even outcomes like obesity. These include data on *food consumption* and the consumption of micro and macro nutrients, which can be obtained from food recall studies. Objective measures of some of the same details can be drawn from biospecimens, including blood and urine, which can be obtained in person along with other health measures including the presence of chronic and acute conditions. NHANES conducts in-person physical examinations, and thus it captures many of these objective biomarkers (using blood and urine draws and a measure of BMI), which offer important insights over and above what one can learn from self-reported measures such as food security and dietary intake.

NHANES's method for obtaining these data also has the advantage over self-reported surveys of providing objective measures of the presence of some conditions that the underinsured and those who rarely visit medical facilities might not know they have. Yet as discussed above, and as is the case with many other datasets, NHANES samples are too small for accurately measuring outcomes by demographic categories (e.g., pregnant women, infants and children, prime-age adults, and the elderly) or by socioeconomic status, and the lack of accurate and well-measured program participation rates limits the ability to compare these health outcomes across programs. There are also limitations due to the lack of state representativeness.

It would be useful if more health-related measures were available that specified program participation and income. This shortcoming stems from the fact that, in most datasets about program participation, all of the characteristics of the respondents are self-reported, so that data on program participation are not accurate. It would be extremely helpful if these health data were linked to administrative program data, as is done in the Census Bureau's Next Generation Data Program and by NCHS, for which Medicaid, Medicare, and Department of Housing and Urban Development (HUD) data are linked to NHANES and NHIS. Broader geographic coverage of food acquisition, nutrition, and food patterns is also important for monitoring.

3.2. ASSESSING THE QUALITY AND COVERAGE OF DATA

In addition to monitoring and surveillance, there are important aspects of the statistical agency role that ERS fills and that crucially need to be continued or expanded. USDA has done an excellent job of examining the quality of proprietary commercial data and some administrative data (Muth, 2018).

This needs to be continued and expanded. It is also crucial to understand who is left out of each form of data, whether that be survey data, proprietary commercial data, or administrative data. Those left out may be firms, such as small ethnic stores or A50 stores. Often outside the scope of surveys or else poorly measured are certain categories of persons, particularly the homeless, certain military personnel, and those living in group quarters. For a different reason, unauthorized immigrants are often left out, because they are less likely to respond to surveys (Capps, Gelatt, and Fix, 2018).

Once data are combined, it is even more important to evaluate the quality of the data integration.[9] This is a major focus of the Next Generation Data Platform (described in Chapter 2, Box 2.2), a cooperative effort between ERS, FNS, and the Census Bureau that has enabled the linking of administrative and survey data to improve models of SNAP eligibility and participation. Whenever time data are merged across sources, it opens the possibility of mismatches or missing matches. Given the reliance on data produced by state and local governments and commercial entities, it is essential to have a process for continually assessing and improving data quality.

In particular, the proprietary sources that FED uses are collected for a variety of clients, and FED is unlikely to be able to dictate items or terms. State and local data, meanwhile, are created for the purposes of running programs and not for ease of integration. For example, a state may have one system for determining WIC eligibility and another unrelated system for reimbursing stores for WIC vouchers. FoodAPS combined several administrative sources of SNAP data, including data from redemptions (ALERT) and from caseload data, but these measures were almost as discordant as the self-reported data from SNAP receipts (Courtemanche, Denteh, and Tchernis, 2019). Even administrative data can have weaknesses stemming from being linked to surveys when it is hard to create individual-level de-identified and linkable Protected Identification Key (PIK) data, such as for new infants who are not yet in the tax data, for highly mobile populations, or when it is hard to assign the administrative records to geographies, as was documented in a 2010 Census planning memo (Rastogi et al, 2010).

3.3. A DATA INFRASTRUCTURE FOR ADDRESSING DESCRIPTIVE AND CAUSAL QUESTIONS

To fulfill its mission, ERS's CFDS must make it possible to answer both descriptive and causal questions. To answer descriptive questions, researchers need access to data to measure the geography of deprivation and nutrition across time, for example, as well as other data to identify correlations

[9] See the discussion of this issue by Robert Moffitt in Appendix B, under the summary of the second meeting.

among demographics, program use, and income. To answer causal questions with observational data, researchers need access to data tracking changes in diet preferences and nutritional knowledge, as well as data on households' ability to use information to make healthful dietary choices.[10] Below, we identify each of the priority areas laid out above and present important questions of each type that remain unanswered but would, ideally, be answerable within the next decade or so with the aid of CFDS.

Food Security

There are multiple research questions regarding food insecurity in the United States. However, to fully address these questions, gaps in currently available information must be filled through upgrades to data sources. Additional questions could be added to surveys, sample sizes could be expanded, and/or often overlooked groups could be better incorporated into data collections with food insecurity components being used by ERS and other researchers and agencies. For example, as covered in Gundersen and Ziliak (2018), there are a host of descriptive research questions, and some causal ones, that deserve investigation. Descriptive questions include these: How is food insecurity distributed within the household? What types of coping mechanisms do low-income but food-secure families use, and what are the effects of those mechanisms? Questions of a more causal nature include

[10]The use of observational data to support causal inferences in the social sciences is not universally accepted as being consistent with best current statistical principles and practices. Some argue that causal inferences are best supported through the use of randomized controlled trials and that observational studies can be misleading and are generally not reliable for this purpose. There is no question that the use of randomized controlled trials has greatly improved our understanding of the efficacy of 'treatments' versus 'controls' in many areas of science and that the causal inferences produced through use of randomized controlled trials are often well-supported. However, it is also the case that randomized controlled trials themselves are sometimes flawed for making causal inferences. For example, Deaton and Cartwright, (2017) point out that "randomization does not equalize everything but the treatment across treatments and controls," and it does not relieve the need by researchers to think about observed or unobserved confounders. Furthermore, perhaps particularly in the social sciences, there are situations where, due to various constraints, randomization of treatment to subject is not feasible (and, in some cases, not ethnical). But the presence of these constraints is not reason to rule out research where causal analyses are nonetheless needed to support policy. Fortunately, as is discussed by Hernán et al. (2008) and others, a number of techniques exist, including various uses of propensity scores, instrumental variables, panel data, differences in differences, and reweighting, that can be used to create treatment effect estimates from observational data that match the results from clinical trials. The techniques used for supporting causal inference in observational studies do require assumptions regarding the adequacy of the set of measured baseline confounders and usefulness of any control groups, but many (although not all) of these assumptions are testable in most observational settings. However, in large studies, the assumptions are often quite reasonable and, in addition, tools for assessing the sensitivity of inferences to the assumptions are available.

these: What are the effects of charitable food assistance programs on food insecurity? What is the causal relationship between food insecurity and health outcomes? How does disability status influence food insecurity? Why is there a declining age gradient in the probability of food insecurity among seniors? How does labor force participation affect food insecurity? What is the impact of changes in the minimum wage on food insecurity? And, what is the impact of the Affordable Care Act on food insecurity?

Regarding the more causal research questions, knowing more than we presently do about patterns of food security over time (within the year) for stable geographies would allow for causal estimates of the effects of school meals. Similarly, being able to make comparisons between food insecurity during the school year and during the summer, a season when program availability is more limited, would be indicative of the role played by policies that remediate food insecurity.

Program Rules about Food Assistance and Other USDA Activities

USDA and the federal government in general have important roles in running food assistance programs. At the same time, state and local governments, which share responsibility with USDA for administering food assistance programs, have many options for deciding what rules individuals, firms, and nonprofits must follow. These options range from deciding which forms of fruits and vegetables—fresh, frozen, or canned—stores must stock in their WIC programs, to choosing the date on which SNAP and WIC benefits are disbursed, to deciding the extent to which applications for SNAP can be made online and where applicants must go to determine their eligibility, to requiring that all schools with a free and reduced lunch certification amount above a certain level participate in the School Breakfast Program. Despite this wide authority and range of options, these state- and locally decided rules are rarely tracked.

As recommended in Chapter 4, creating a database for each of the other programs analogous to the databases currently tracking SNAP options for eligibility and disbursal would advance research estimating associations and causal effects, on a number of topics that now happen only slowly and haphazardly. Research would also be empowered by the tracking of rules for firms and the geography of those assessing eligibility and providing benefits. Constructing these databases would enable the study of program use and eligibility by persons, of program participation by firms, and the extent to which the locations of government entities determining eligibility affect take-up by individuals.

Tracking the rules described in the previous section is the first step in calculating whether individuals are potentially eligible to participate in the food assistance programs. Eligibility will vary for specific members of the population depending on income and assets and, at times, other factors. High-quality panel data on people and firms are also needed to be able to use the eligibility rules described above to predict whether households, individuals, or firms are potentially eligible to participate in the programs.

Moreover, it is also necessary to maintain high-quality administrative data on where program participants live and where they spend their benefits to understand how programs are used and who among those eligible takes up programs. Incomplete take-up is thought to be a product of stigma, transactions costs, lack of information, and the cognitive burden of poverty. Eligibility and participation data would allow for comprehensive examinations of the targeting of these programs and help promote better understanding of issues pertaining to take-up. All of this is important for understanding whether programs are effectively on the margin targeting the most needy, as behavioral science would suggest be done, or whether they are on the margin reaching the least needy among participants. Recent research suggests this is not uniform across programs and eligibility and outreach efforts (e.g., Deshpande and Li, 2017; Finkelstein and Notowidigdo, 2019).

Ideally, assistance programs should reach those most in need; in other words, they should be "well-targeted." When this is the case, households that are less-in-need (in terms of the goals of the program) would be less likely to participate, including households with incomes near the eligibility threshold and/or incomes that are likely to exceed the threshold in the near future. In addition, for households with characteristics reflecting higher asset levels (including human capital), the benefits they receive from food assistance may not exceed the total costs when one considers stigma and transaction costs.

A concern emerges, though, when households with higher levels of need do not enter a program. In many cases, this may happen because the costs to enter the program may be perceived to be higher than the benefits or involve some other dimension than can be addressed by policy changes. For example, many vulnerable households may not have information about the program or, even if they are aware of it, may find that the administrative hurdles to entering the program are too high. By reducing these costs—such as the cost of obtaining information or the costs of the application and recertification process—programs may be able to increase participation rates.[11]

In the case of SNAP, this difference between types of nonreceipt is evident when one looks at the over-age-60 group in comparison with the

[11]For analyses of SNAP churn, see articles by Ribar and Edelhoch (2008) and Mills et al. (2014).

age-40-to-60 group. For the former, the low participation rates can largely be explained by observed characteristics while, for the latter, it is not clear why the participation rates are low (Gundersen and Ziliak, 2008). The geographic and time detail discussed above can provide insights into the reasons for nonparticipation and, in particular, whether there are ways to increase participation among the more vulnerable.

While some of these administrative data, made available with limited geographic detail (such as the state level for the WIC PC data by FNS) are already used by individual researchers or by the Census Bureau and others, there is no comprehensive set of such data spanning all states and programs. Further, simply tracking the location of WIC clinics, schools participating in school meals, SNAP offices, and other program delivery and eligibility determination sites would facilitate important research on program take-up, especially for the smaller programs that are not well studied, such as CACFP. Knowing where potentially eligible stores are located and which stores participate would allow researchers to model store choices regarding program participation and track where programs are hard to access. Knowing the geography of nonprofit school, clinic, and CACFP participation choices will also be useful.

Maintaining accessible administrative data on the programs from all 50 states and the District of Columbia would also improve statistics on take-up and poverty, as long as there is also a suitable source of data on the full population to determine who is eligible for the programs. These data could be used to augment Census or other measures of self-reported program participation if linkages from administrative sources to possible sources of the full population are robust. While a large number of states currently share at least one source of state-run program data with the Census, a much smaller group shares WIC, TANF, and SNAP information. To the extent that these states are not randomly sharing their data but may have different populations, evidence generated from analysis using these states' data may not generalize to the whole nation. Expansion of the ERS/Census Bureau's Next Generation Data Platform would enable researchers to study the interactions between USDA programs and other programs, if the data were made widely available to outside researchers.

The Food Environment

It would be useful to have descriptive information to track changes in the retail food environment—for example, the rise of dollar stores, the locations of ethnic food markets, the growth of delivery services through venues such as Amazon, Costco, Walmart, and meal-kits. Little is known, even descriptively, about the many small nonchain stores lacking point-of-service technology where low-income individuals and families often shop and redeem food assistance vouchers.[12] Cuffey and Beatty (2019) suggest that about 11 percent of SNAP redemptions in Minneapolis occur at such stores. Tying these data to data covering other sources of food, such as restaurants (with associated information about the dietary quality of offerings), schools, day care facilities, and providers of free or subsidized meals would help complete the picture of the food landscape. Combining existing scanner data with data on stores participating in SNAP (using the Store Tracking and Redemption System or STARS) and WIC (TIPS[13]) would help researchers to track smaller stores and would augment existing sources such as TD LINX.[14]

Next, we turn to some causal questions, which place even greater demands on the underlying data needed to answer them. Repeated cross-sections of food environment data are needed to evaluate geographically targeted policies, such as those addressing poor food environments by proposing taxes on sugar-sweetened beverages, or the Healthy Food Financing Initiative, which sought to improve access to healthy foods by helping to cover some of the costs of setting up grocery stores. It is not easy for many researchers to access to data with detailed geography on food intake or food acquisition in order to study how such local policies might affect outcomes. Other data sources, such as scanner data may be expensive, lack coverage, or are unable to link to fine geographies. Government survey alternatives, such as NHANES, are constrained by limited geographic coverage.

In addition to the food environment, information on other components of the geography facing low-income households would be relevant. As an example, high housing prices are often a constraint on the ability of households to be food secure. By overlaying housing prices onto the information noted above, this could be investigated. As another example, in some parts of the country there have been increases (or proposed increases) in the minimum wage. The impact of these changes on food insecurity and other food outcomes are ambiguous and, therefore, including this in a comprehensive overview of the food environment could be useful.

---

[12]FNS recently published results of a survey of small SNAP retail stores about their ability to adopt scanning technology if needed in the future. See https://fns-prod.azureedge.net/sites/default/files/resource-files/SNAPScanner-Capability.pdf.

[13]TIP Data Collection is intended to provide FNS and WIC state agencies with "an annual dataset that can be used to assess State agencies' compliance with WIC vendor management requirements and estimate State agencies' progress in eliminating fraud, waste, and abuse." See https://www.federalregister.gov/documents/2018/03/21/2018-05704/agency-information-collection-activities-proposed-collection-comment-request-special-supplemental.

[14]As described in Chapter 2, STARS from FNS and TDLinx from Nielsen have been used to assess characteristics of the food retail environment, such as the locations and characteristics of food retailers and restaurants.

Consumption

Descriptive data enable researchers to track the evolution of new product attributes and novel food characteristics. For causal research, however, more is needed. For example, it would be helpful to be able to track changes in diet preferences and in people's knowledge of and ability to use information to make healthful dietary choices. Yet there are holes in our knowledge of food consumption preferences and the choices of some urban residents and very-low-income households, because these populations are insufficiently represented in Nielsen and IRI data sources and because errors are made in recording in general (e.g., Einav, Leibtag, and Nevo, 2010).

Other questions that could be addressed with more data include whether new products arise because of changes in preferences or, alternatively, because of technological change. Data tracking of net product characteristics would also enable more focused analyses of the role of information provision from the federal government, private sources (advertising), and other public sources in changing food demand. This is particularly important for understanding possible market failures caused by imperfect information that is linked to food choices. These market failures arise due to changes in nutrition science and our understanding of what a healthful diet is, because food is a "credence good," that is, a good whose quality consumers cannot assess until after they have consumed it, and also because the provision of information provision can shift the salience of attributes of food, such as "healthful" or "organic."

Prices

Descriptively, detailed price data, as discussed above, would permit analysis of the relative affordability of different kinds of foods, healthful and otherwise, across time and over space. Detailed price data would also allow researchers to study causal questions, such as how differences in the real value of SNAP and WIC benefits affect food acquisition and consumption and subsequent health and other outcomes. While there has been some research on this topic (e.g., Gregory and Coleman-Jensen, 2013; Courtemanche, Denteh, and Tchernis, 2019; Bronchetti, Christensen, and Hoynes, 2019), it has used data aggregated at perhaps too high a level, such as the county or regional level, and it has depended on too limited a set of price indexes. By incorporating the relative prices of non-store sources of food helps researchers to better understand the impacts of food prices.

Time Use

Insofar as people often eat while engaged in other tasks, it can be difficult to track eating as a "primary task." Monitoring eating as a secondary activity is important and has been enabled by the Eating and Health Module of the ATUS. Continuing to track these important time-use patterns requires an ongoing commitment to this sort of data collection. It also would be useful to know more about how people trade off their time with other resources across various income flows coming into people's homes. This could be done, for example, when considering where and how people shop and the extent to which they purchase near-ready foods, such as frozen meals, versus raw ingredients. Lastly, the various food plans make assumptions about peoples' ability and willingness to prepare food from scratch. It would be useful to consider time concerns when creating the food plans.

Food-Related Health Measurement

Larger samples of these health outcomes that span more detailed geographic areas would permit researchers to better study the effects of policy and other determinants of food choice on health and nutrition outcomes, beyond the most basic outcome of food security. They would also permit better monitoring of health and nutrition and program use. Combining health data with nationally representative data that accurately measure use of programs and income flows would allow the study of questions such as how policy affects programs, food choice, and health.

We also note that many useful projects have been conducted with data collected by other agencies. Better coordination with other agencies might help avoid such problems as the failure of important surveys to collect or merge administrative data on programs, as happened with the Early Childhood Longitudinal Study, Kindergarten Class of 2010–2011, where receipt of school meals was not reported at the individual level. One example of such a useful link is provided with NHANES's and NHIS's links to Medicaid, Medicare, and other administrative data.

Although extensive work has been done on the impact of food insecurity on current health status (for a review, see Gundersen and Ziliak, 2018), the longer-term impacts are still an open question. This is primarily due to not having a consistent set of food insecurity questions on any panel dataset. PSID included questions from 1997 to 2003, but due to lack of funding those questions were removed until 2015. The continued inclusion of these questions on PSID would be welcome, as it would enable an understanding of issues such as how food insecurity in childhood is transmitted into long-term health and human capital outcomes as adults and whether food insecurity is transmitted across generations.

3.4. CONCLUSION

In this chapter, strengths and some gaps in the statistical system's coverage of consumer food and nutrition choices and associated outcomes have been laid out. In some cases, identified in Chapter 4, these are domains where the CFDS does and should provide data to enable the study of descriptive and causal questions. We have also discussed the important role of the FED in serving ERS's role as a statistical agency. We have included the specific questions we think are required to provide evidence for policy makers and the public alike so that they have the information necessary to make decisions that will make the country a better place in 2050.

But new issues are sure to arise. We urge the Food Economics Division to keep the following issues in mind going forward, toward a time when, should current demographic trends continue, the country is sure to be more racially and ethnically diverse. The country is also likely to have more mixed family structures, including more cohabitation, single-parent households, and multi-generational households, varying concentrations of poverty, and mixed immigration status. For example, shared custody may have implications for defining an economic unit of people who eat together. Separately from demographic changes, changing food technology and preferences may alter the shelf stability of many foods, with implications for the types of storage needed to store foods. Tastes are set by early exposure to specific kinds of foods, and programs can affect this.

All of these evolving issues require a forward-looking mindset and a cohesive agenda in data collection. In the next chapter, we lay out a series of recommendations to advance the CFDS in a way that would fill a number of the data and knowledge gaps identified here.

4

Strategies to Strengthen the Infrastructure of a Consumer Food Data System

4.1. DESIRABLE CHARACTERISTICS OF A CONSUMER FOOD DATA SYSTEM

This panel was charged with reviewing the Consumer Food Data System (CFDS) program for the Economic Research Service (ERS) and providing guidance for its advancement over the next 10 years. As part of this charge, the panel was asked "to identify data gaps and to anticipate how evolving policy priorities may affect data needs." Recognizing that the objective of the CFDS program is to advance understanding of food acquisition, behavior, and outcomes, the panel identified characteristics of a CFDS that is effective and useful for research and policy purposes. These include comprehensiveness, representativeness, timeliness, openness, flexibility, accuracy, suitability, and fiscal responsibility. These characteristics are aspirational for the CFDS *in toto* and may not be met in any one data resource.

Comprehensiveness

A data system that is effective for monitoring the levels and trends in food behaviors and outcomes and for identifying the effects of public programs and policies on those behaviors requires comprehensive data. These data need to come from a variety of sources and to span multiple topics. Surveys are useful in documenting socioeconomic factors that affect food behaviors and outcomes, such as family/household structure, age, gender, race, education, employment, income, health status, (nonfood) consumption, wealth, time use, and geography, among others. Traditionally surveys have also been the main source for data on program participation within the Supplemental Nutrition Assistance Program (SNAP), Special Supplemental Nutrition Program for Women, Infants, and Children (WIC), Temporary Assistance for Needy Families (TANF), and other safety net programs.

However, surveys have been decreasingly reliable for such analyses, owing to rising rates of nonresponse. Further, surveys suffer from respondent error in reporting program participation. (Meyer, Mok, and Sullivan, 2015; Bollinger et al., 2019). When administrative data are linked to surveys, the combination provides improved accuracy relative to surveys alone for measurement of and the evaluation of transfer programs (concerning both participation and benefit levels). Independent of their linkage to surveys, administrative data are useful for purposes of general program monitoring, as well as for certain forms of evaluation such as "leaver" studies.

Because consumer food choices respond to economic, policy, and environmental incentives, an effective food data system also requires access to comprehensive information on food prices, food policies, food outlets, and the spectrum of food choices within those outlets. Some granular data on prices, outlets, and choices can be obtained from surveys of markets, directly provided by food vendors, or from third-party private aggregators such as Nielsen and IRI. Information on food policies at the federal, state, and local level is essential to understanding the constraints and options facing potential recipients and thus is useful in nonexperimental evaluations of food assistance programs. An exemplar of the latter is the SNAP Policy Database, currently collected by ERS.

Representativeness

Data on food behaviors and outcomes are most useful if they are representative of the U.S. population, both nationally and at component aggregations such as states. National-level representativeness is needed to accurately assess aggregate levels and trends. Because many food and health programs and policies vary across states, a data system that is of adequate size and representative of the diversity of households at the state level is desirable. Given ERS's important focus on rural areas as well as the rest of the country, representativeness along the urban-rural continuum is also desirable. Household surveys that are representative at the substate level are generally cost-prohibitive; however, administrative and scanner data are generally of high value-added at the substate level owing to their very large samples, and administrative data also do not suffer from coverage or nonresponse issues within the population of program participants.

One concern about extant scanner and some privately collected commercial data is their lack of coverage in rural areas. Thus, having a data system that also reflects the food environment for rural and other hard-to-reach populations, in addition to reflecting the rest of the country, should be a goal of an effective CFDS.

In addition to providing comprehensive data, an effective data system would sample the same households, firms, or geographies repeatedly over time. Ideally these data would be longitudinal in that they follow the same households or firms over time without substantial attrition, but repeated cross-sections of households or firms collected from the same geographic areas over time are also well suited for causal research designs with observational data. Administrative and scanner data lend themselves to longitudinal data formats, since individuals and firms can be readily linked over time with unique IDs (e.g., by Social Security number, Employer Identification Number, or proprietary identifiers). Repeated household measures are preferred when there is not substantial attrition or nonresponse. Nevertheless, much can be learned from repeated cross-sectional data, for example by exploiting changes in the policy environment across states and over time. Whether panel or repeated cross-section, the data are most effective for monitoring and evaluation if the questionnaire's content and structure are stable over time.

Timeliness

To have maximum program and policy impact, an effective data system needs to collect data at regular intervals, and its data metrics must be consistent over time to allow accurate tracking of trends. The interval of data collection will differ depending on the programmatic need. Many monitoring functions, including the measurement of program participation in food assistance in SNAP, WIC, and school meal programs, require data at a monthly frequency, while other monitoring, including the tracking of health and nutrition outcomes such as diabetes and obesity, is more slow-moving and can be sufficiently handled by annual data collection. Many evaluations of behavioral outcomes are also effectively conducted with annual data. Thus, the minimum interval for collecting data on the program policy environment is annual.

Openness

A data system is effective if it is open and accessible to the public and to the policy and research communities, although the degree of openness should vary based on the "need to know." Because the programs and data are collected with taxpayer funds, some data used to monitor program policies and participation, as well as health and dietary outcomes, should be readily accessible to the general public for the sake of transparency concerning program reach and operations. Generally, such data are currently publicly available, aggregated at the county, state, or national level over time.

For some nonexperimental monitoring and evaluations of food behaviors and outcomes, a de-identified individual-level dataset (at the household or firm level) to which the public has open access for research purposes is desirable. To be most effective, such data should contain identifying geographic information but restricted to a level sufficient to protect respondent confidentiality, such as state of residence or, in some cases, county of residence. This approach permits merging the data with state-level or county-level information from other sources (e.g., the SNAP Policy Database or the Bureau of Labor Statistics' state and county unemployment rates), which is standard practice in nonexperimental evaluations. Some monitoring and evaluations of food and health outcomes require access to more granular geographic data, such as latitude and longitude of location or the Census block or tract level.

Still other research requires access to the individual or firm IDs, for example to link survey data to administrative data, or else across administrative data sources. In such cases, policies and procedures are needed (and indeed are in place) to ensure that access to the restricted data is limited to qualified researchers while protecting privacy. One model for accomplishing this is that of the Federal Statistical Research Data Centers (FSRDCs)—a partnership between federal statistical agencies and leading research institutions in which secure facilities provide authorized access to restricted-use microdata for statistical purposes only.[1] Further examples were proposed by the bipartisan U.S. Commission on Evidence-Based Policymaking.[2]

ERS offered an alternative to the FSRDC system for those who wished to use restricted versions of National Household Food Acquisition and Purchase Survey (FoodAPS), but access to the IRI data linked to the FoodAPS would have required signing an indemnity clause, which is forbidden for many researchers at state universities, and thus would have failed the open-access goal of a desirable data system. Policies and procedures for access to restricted versions of the various datasets should be established in cooperation with representatives from the user community.

Human subjects' protections and privacy rules sometimes limit the way data may be shared. Hence, the CFDS should be conceived in a modular

[1] See https://www.census.gov/fsrdc.

[2] The Commission was a 15-member group of experts charged by the U.S. Congress and the president with examining how government could better use its existing data sources to provide high-quality evidence for policy and government decision making. The Commission was created in March 2016 by the Evidence-Based Policymaking Commission Act (P.L. 114-140), legislation jointly filed by Speaker of the House Paul Ryan (R-WI) and Senator Patty Murray (D-WA) https://www.congress.gov/bill/114th-congress/house-bill/1831.

fashion, with each type of data being shared in the most open manner consistent with human subjects' protections and privacy rules. Personal data are protected under state and local laws, which require agencies to prevent unauthorized access through security controls on the information technology systems that process and store data. Privacy protections also extend beyond security controls. Agencies decide who can use program data (e.g., employees, contractors, and research partners) and for what purposes (e.g., program evaluation, program improvement, research, and compliance reporting). To support uniform, secure access to administrative data, ERS can provide interpretation of federal statutes and data management protocols to streamline data comparisons and linkages. ERS can also provide guidance on reducing privacy risks in published data aggregates and reports, including disclosure avoidance tools and checklists.

Data access should not be limited to groups with close connections to USDA. For example, Nielsen data must be protected, but its price data in aggregate form is shared in the Quarterly Food-at-Home Price Index constructed by ERS. Similarly, FoodAPS data are shared through a data enclave with NORC at the University of Chicago,[3] but they are also available in less detail through public-use files.

Access should also be timely and not require a huge financial burden, thus permitting their use by a broader set of researchers, including those with expertise in economics, nutrition, health policy, geographic information systems, and clinical care. Of course, the USDA ERS staff are perhaps the most expert users of some of the data in the CFDS, given their role in creating it, but facilitating more outside access would also be useful for science and policy.

Flexibility

Ideally, investments in food and consumer data go on to support (i) research applications that were planned in advance, (ii) unanticipated applications generated by a broad, entrepreneurial, and inventive community of research users, and (iii) efforts to evaluate unanticipated changes in policy and in food retail markets.

ERS's development and inclusion of the Household Food Security Module as a supplement to the Current Population Survey (CPS; prompted by a congressional request) was crucial in that it unleashed an entirely new research and policy agenda. This has allowed the research and policy communities to plan, years in advance, for reports on food insecurity to coincide with the annual release of the data. Another example of planned use was the design of FoodAPS, which allowed researchers to study how the

[3]See http://www.norc.org/Research/Capabilities/Pages/data-enclave.aspx.

SNAP issuance cycle affects food acquisition or diet quality (Smith et al., 2016; Kuhn, 2018; Whiteman, Chrisinger, and Hillie, 2018).

However, in some cases new ideas or policies have emerged that were unanticipated. Similarly, new forms of food acquisition are emerging, such as online delivery. Thus, a desirable data system must be elastic to respond to such innovations.

Accuracy

Accurate measurement and reporting are the foundation of effective evidence-based policy making, so a desirable data system is one that seeks continuous quality checking and improvement. For surveys this entails, among other things, minimizing nonresponse to questions or to the survey itself as well as minimizing reporting error. Linking survey data to administrative data offers the prospect of better measurement of household participation in assistance programs when links are of high quality, but administrative data, which generally originate from state governments, are not devoid of measurement error. Scanner data on persons and establishments, while rich in granularity, also suffer from underreporting of certain items and often lack coverage of certain populations, notably low-income people and those residing in rural areas. They also often fail to include all the outcomes of interest. Thus, a program of ongoing studies to assess the quality, coverage, and comprehensiveness of surveys, administrative records, and scanner data is needed.

Suitability

While some CFDS purposes are descriptive, others require cause-and-effect inference. The CFDS should anticipate the implications that the desire for achieving causal results may have in its data design. These include the collection and sharing of policy variables for use in executing quasi-experimental designs, the use of program data (or surveys that include nonparticipants) as sampling frames for potential program evaluations using random-assignment experimental research designs, and the use of administrative data to improve inference based on faulty self-reports. They also include the use of longitudinal data for statistical analyses that control for certain types of time-constant and location-constant confounding variables in estimating causal effects, or the use of other econometric approaches offering causal insight (e.g., instrumental variables, Regression Discontinuity Design). They also include the curation of data to maintain version control and enable archiving to support replication.

Features of a (nonexperimental) data system that facilitate strong causal research designs include (i) the provision of sampling frames through administrative data that can be used for random assignment or survey purposes; (ii) the provision of comparison data that are nationally representative for use in understanding the study populations through nonexperimental evaluations; (iii) integration with policy information as explanatory variables (as has been emphasized in the SNAP rules parts of this report); (iv) longitudinal or panel structures for use in fixed-effects models that control for unobserved time-constant confounding variables; and (v) inclusion of appropriate administrative data on program participation linked with nationally or regionally representative survey or administrative data on the population of potentially eligible persons.

Fiscal Responsibility

Taxpayer dollars should be spent wisely. This is especially true today in an era of tightening statistical agency budgets. The CFDS should maximize the research value of federal dollars invested in the data system through its combined impact on improved program monitoring, improved monitoring of the nutritional status, food security, and health of the population, and strengthened ability to conduct research estimating the causal linkages between programs and outcomes. ERS's CFDS strategy should encompass both investments in special-purpose surveys and initiatives to enhance the research value of administrative data, survey data, and other sources of data already being collected for nonresearch purposes, such as proprietary commercial data. Investment into data products should be diversified to allow for unexpected research directions.

Achieving the above-described characteristics in a data system to support food and nutrition research requires taking a multipronged approach involving survey, administrative, and commercial data.[4] The 20th century survey-centric federal statistical system is at a crossroads: Declining response rates have led to surveys becoming more costly and the resulting data possibly becoming less accurate or generalizable, while lower-burden complementary or substitute administrative and proprietary data sources have emerged. The report of the Commission on Evidence-Based Policymaking (2017) lays out many of the challenges and advantages of combining different types of data. Among them are (i) the changes in consumer food shopping modes (e.g., increased food shopping online), which will likely continue to elevate the importance to researchers of nonsurvey data sources such as proprietary data and administrative data; and (ii) assessing the quality, coverage, and representativeness or generalizability of these non-survey data sources, which will be increasingly important.

[4]As articulated by Larimore et al. (2018), this has been a stated goal of ERS for several years.

Broadly, the challenge is to put each type of data source—surveys, administrative data, and proprietary data—to its best use. Administrative data are best for accurately measuring the use of programs. Survey data can provide rich information on outcomes such as nutrition and health measures while also providing nationally or regionally representative population samples with which to merge the administrative data. Proprietary data are best for high-frequency measures, such as purchases in real time, which would be prohibitively expensive and perhaps infeasible to track with surveys. As discussed in Chapter 2, administrative data can be strengthened, coordinated, and integrated with survey data and put to better use than they now are; similarly, proprietary data could be used more extensively, if made more accessible. Sections 4.2–4.6 detail our ideas for ways ERS can move forward as it continues the development of its multipronged data system combining surveys, proprietary data, and administrative data. We discuss each of these separately, as well as the importance of integration.

A consumer food data system, such as that maintained by ERS, contains information at the individual, household, and firm level from surveys, administrative data systems, and commercial proprietary data that are representative and accurate at the national, state, and local levels, as demanded by the purposes to which they are put. These data, collected from governmental and nongovernmental agencies and organizations, ideally at regularly scheduled intervals, cover food acquisitions, food security, food prices, food assistance program participation and eligibility, demographics, and health and economic outcomes. Data are needed for monitoring purposes on a regular basis, to allow comparisons over time and to support causal research. Some purposes require data that are repeated cross-sections or longitudinal at the individual, household, or firm level.

4.2. SURVEY COMPONENTS OF THE CFDS

As articulated in Chapter 2, surveys have long been a central data source in consumer food and nutrition research. Survey data provide insight into household- and person-level variables about outcomes that frequently are missing in administrative data. Some surveys have the advantage of linkage between food-related variables and diverse other variables of interest. While surveys are comparatively expensive on a per-observation basis, in the past they have provided researchers with representative samples. Nevertheless, this strength is challenged by increasing difficulties with participation rates, the high respondent burden in some surveys, increased misreporting of important variables such as program participation and income, and lack of timeliness.

Below we touch on the need for some data sources that measure the population at risk of specific outcomes or measure participation in programs, which often come from surveys. In this section, we provide guidance for future investments in survey data and then offer more detailed recommendations for selected important data sources, especially FoodAPS. We also offer recommendations for survey data for monitoring food security, for linkages with nutrition data in the National Health and Nutrition Examination Survey (NHANES), for time use, and for program evaluation. Taken together, the recommendations in this chapter create a vision for survey data that, by comparison with current practice, is somewhat smaller in scope, somewhat higher in cost per observation, more focused on selected applications that cannot be served by other data sources, and more integrated with administrative and commercial data.

General Findings and Recommendations about Surveys

Surveys will continue to be important to statistical agencies for the foreseeable future. They provide household- and individual-level data that cannot always be acquired through other means. Due to increasing concerns with data quality and response rates, survey investments must keep up with current best practices in survey design and implementation (Groves et al., 2009).

RECOMMENDATION 4.1: A key task for the Consumer Food Data System is to assess the quality of survey data across sources and over time. This should be done by linking the surveys to auxiliary sources in order to check sample records. For example, work comparing population totals and individual reports of program participation can be done by comparing survey totals to administrative totals and comparing self-reports to administrative records. The level of missing data and the characteristics of those missing data should be catalogued.

USDA should anticipate in advance that investments satisfying these current best practices will be expensive on a per-observation basis. This implies limits on the total growth of federal investments in traditional stand-alone surveys.

RECOMMENDATION 4.2: To make effective use of limited resources for survey investments, the U.S. Department of Agriculture should further exploit both administrative data sources and commercial data sources for applications wherein they can be effectively used.

For example, whereas survey data sources have in the past been an important source for understanding determinants of program participation and for research on entry and exit dynamics (Mabli and Ohls, 2012), the CFDS should plan for increased use of administrative data and reduced use of survey-only data for these purposes (Ribar and Swann, 2014).

In some cases, the expense of survey data collection may require USDA to focus on a few high-priority research applications, recognizing that other desired research topics cannot be addressed with survey investments that are feasible, given budgetary constraints. Two examples of high-priority topics that will continue to require survey investments are the monitoring of household food security outcomes and measurements of the impact of nutrition assistance programs on food insecurity and dietary intakes.

As discussed in section 4.6, blended approaches, in which survey data are combined with administrative and commercial data, hold great promise for creating added value and lowering costs per observation. This can be achieved through use of blending in frame development, sample unit screening, edits and imputations, augmenting by joining additional content, and modeling (e.g., small area estimation and simulations).

Recommendations for FoodAPS

FoodAPS, which is sponsored by ERS and the Food and Nutrition Services (FNS), is currently the most visible component of the CFDS. As described in detail in Chapter 2, FoodAPS is designed to generate data on household food acquisitions for different populations, particularly low-income households, including food-insecure households and those participating in SNAP and other government programs. By collecting data on all the places where people purchase and acquire food, FoodAPS was an improvement on previous options about acquisition of food for home and away from home.

USDA invested heavily in independent assessments of FoodAPS to better understand data quality. These assessments reflect a strong emphasis on accuracy, one of the key desirable data system characteristics noted earlier in this chapter. USDA also invested in understanding the strengths and weaknesses in FoodAPS from the perspective of researchers and data users (Wilde and Ismail, 2018). Results of these assessments and activities are reviewed in detail in Chapter 2. In a bid to introduce FoodAPS to the research community, and consistent with the desirable data system characteristic of openness, ERS and FNS also underwrote numerous projects by external researchers selected through grant competitions hosted by the National Bureau of Economic Research and the University of Kentucky Center for Poverty Research.

FoodAPS will remain useful for carrying out the descriptive and monitoring functions concerning overall food acquisition. Because the greatest strength of FoodAPS for research and policy is in its capacity to generate descriptive and monitoring information on food acquisition habits, which likely change slowly over time, and because it is an expensive survey, it is not practical to envision it as an annual or even semiannual program. That said, there is clear value to conducting the survey on a regular basis, as doing so allows it to contribute to the construction of stylized facts for the monitoring function of CFDS. There are benefits to using a fixed and predictable schedule (e.g., as the Census Bureau does with the Economic Census). Doing so may generate efficiencies and predictability by creating a regular staffing cycle, which is important for ERS in managing the data system and not having other valuable components of the CFDS suffer when FoodAPS's resource demands are high.

RECOMMENDATION 4.3: The National Household Food Acquisition and Purchase Survey should be conducted on a regular schedule, such as once every 5 years.

The move to a regular schedule will also allow ERS to plan for the integration of new data sources such as administrative data on multiple programs. This aspect of data coordination should be improved, and likely would be in the presence of fixed periodicity and use of similar data acquisition modules. The ordered planning cycle would facilitate continual process improvement and institutional memory about how a national survey is conducted. This approach would also avoid paying the fixed costs of conducting new surveys at uneven time intervals. At the same time, consistent questions over time also improve the usefulness of these data by, for example, allowing for comparability across assessments of time trends.

To the extent that FoodAPS is intended to support research beyond monitoring of food acquisitions and related outcomes, such as longitudinal and causal research, planners can learn from other surveys that match a sample to longitudinal administrative data both retrospectively and prospectively. For example, the Survey of Income and Program Participation (SIPP) Social Security Administration (SSA) Supplement linked data support studies on program participation and take-up for programs administered by the SSA that are critical for government and academic policy simulation and evaluation. CPS linked to longitudinal Social Security payroll tax records permits analyses of earnings over the life course (inequality, volatility, mobility) that would not be possible with the repeated cross-sections of the CPS alone.

Related, future iterations of FoodAPS could sample from the same geographical units—the same primary sampling units (PSUs)—to create a repeated cross-sectional design. This would permit researchers to combine cross-PSU over time changes in socioeconomic conditions, policy choices, and the built environment to assess how economic, policy, and environmental factors affect food acquisitions and related outcomes collected in FoodAPS, which is a method employed in many quasi-experimental research studies.

RECOMMENDATION 4.4: The National Household Food Acquisition and Purchase Survey should be reviewed across a set of design dimensions for future iterations. Along with linkages to extant administrative records from other federal and state statistical agencies, the review should assess the efficacy of sampling from the same set of primary sampling units over time to facilitate more rigorous monitoring and evaluation functions.

FoodAPS has been effective in getting appropriate samples of SNAP recipients because of its use of a dual frame, with one frame composed of SNAP recipients and the other of everyone else. However, it has been expensive to get enough eligible nonparticipants in the sample to make detailed comparisons with participants. It may be more efficient in future rounds of FoodAPS to go even further in the use of administrative and commercial data to create the initial frame, which would cut the cost of screening the non-SNAP participant samples. An example of this approach is the National Survey of Children's Health done by the Census Bureau. Another example is the Health and Retirement Study funded by the National Institute on Aging but with data collection by the University of Michigan Survey Research Center. Future rounds of FoodAPS could consider these alternative techniques. In addition, due to great interest in oversampling WIC households, program planners should consider including a sufficient sample of WIC recipients (and eligible nonrecipients) using a frame of WIC administrative data.

More broadly, the FoodAPS team can seek and apply best practices in survey design to reduce the burden on respondents and overall costs while improving data quality. Examples include: (1) using adaptive survey design and tailoring the survey operations to optimize participation and using data to monitor when to change course; (2) using auxiliary data in frame development; (3) screening (e.g., generating adequate samples of households with incomes above/below program cutoffs); and (4) mixed-mode designs. The survey design should incorporate greater use of administrative and proprietary data in imputing missing data, adding content depth, and adding longitudinal content.

Broadly speaking, FoodAPS should not be seen as a stand-alone centerpiece of the CFDS, but rather as a key contributor to a system that also incorporates other complementary data sources. Importantly, FoodAPS should not be prioritized over other major initiatives that are funded by ERS or for which ERS plays a supervisory role such as the food security modules in the CPS, NHIS, NHANES, and PSID, the Next Generation

Data Platform, person and firm-level scanner data, SNAP Policy Database, and efforts to document strengths and weaknesses of all the data products. Given the response rate and participant burden challenges facing not just FoodAPS, but surveys across the entire statistical system, it is always important to look for opportunities to scale back the length of the survey instruments and simplify the data collection procedures. Indeed, along with increasing accuracy, this has been a major motivation behind ERS's integration of external data sources for food products linked with Universal Product Code (UPC) codes or retail receipt coding. Statistical agencies today are envisioning a future in which there will be much more blending of mixed data types. As explicitly recommended in section 4.3 below, when a major survey such as FoodAPS is designed, the role of administrative data or other data types in the overall design and estimation strategy should be considered, including the coverage, quality, timeliness, accessibility, and cost of those data. This attention to total error in the mixed data system broadens the total survey approach that ERS already practices in its survey data collection.

Use of Survey Modules

USDA will no doubt continue to collect data using the modules already strategically placed on other surveys (the current use of such modules is documented in Chapter 2). Vehicles such as the Flexible Consumer Behavior Survey and the Eating and Health Module, among others, exploit the strengths of surveys and take advantage of the explanatory covariates contained in other data collections.

RECOMMENDATION 4.5: ERS should advocate for continued funding of data collection, and research on food security should be treated as a high priority in the Current Population Survey, National Health Interview Survey, National Health and Nutrition Examination Survey, and the Panel Study of Income Dynamics.

As discussed in Chapter 2, food security is emphasized in many ERS and FNS-funded modules, in part because the agency is mandated to collect data on food adequacy and has done so on a regular basis for many years.[5] The Food Security Supplement to the CPS was prompted by the National

[5]An earlier Committee on National Statistics report (NRC, 2006) shifted the focus of household surveys away from hunger and toward the measurement and monitoring of food insecurity. Hunger, the panel concluded, is "a separate concept from food insecurity . . . [and] an important potential consequence of food insecurity" and it is "an individual and not a household construct."

Nutrition Monitoring and Related Research Act of 1990.[6] The full module of the CPS contains 18 items, with both 30-day and 12-month reference periods. The National Health Interview Survey (NHIS) contains a shorter, 10-item set of adult-focused questions pertaining to the prior 30 days (as does FoodAPS). NHANES and the PSID contain the full 18-item module for the prior 12 months. The 18-item module with a 12-month reference period is preferred both because of the importance of monitoring child-specific exposure to food insecurity and because most of the survey questions on program participation, income, consumption, health, and other domains refer to the prior 12 months (or prior calendar year) and beyond.[7]

RECOMMENDATION 4.6: The Economic Research Service should recommend that the 10-item, 30-day measure currently used in the National Household Food Acquisition and Purchase Survey and the National Health Interview Survey should be replaced in future iterations of these surveys with the 18-item, 12-month module.

Another key set of measures for monitoring the healthfulness of American diets concerns food intake. Currently, 2-day food intake is measured in NHANES. Yet, for many purposes, the sample sizes are too small to allow meaningful policy analysis.[8] The most direct way to alleviate this shortcoming would be to financially support the Centers for Disease Control and Prevention, which sponsors the NHANES, to expand the sample size of individuals whose intake is measured on NHANES.

4.3. OPPORTUNITIES FROM AND CHALLENGES WITH EXPANDING USE OF ADMINISTRATIVE DATA

This report calls for a balance of survey and administrative data sources, as well as an integration of commercial data (as discussed in section 4.4 below). It is well recognized that a data system sometimes requires surveys to measure outcome variables, such as food intake, and to achieve representativeness of the entire population (rather than, for example, just program participants). Moreover, as described in Chapter 2, administrative data have both strengths and limitations just as survey data do. Several

[6] See https://fns-prod.azureedge.net/sites/default/files/FSGuide.pdf.

[7] Schmidt et al. (2016) present evidence of an inconsistency in how the social safety net affects food insecurity, finding a significant attenuation with the 12-month measure and no effect using the 30-day measure. They conjecture that the difference may be due to the differential timing of transfer-program measurement (12 month) and the 30-day measure.

[8] For example, one expert panel (NASEM, 2017b) determined that the sample sizes of pregnant women on and not on WIC were so small that the panel felt they did not support robust statistical comparisons.

institutions have carefully defined ways of assessing the quality of administrative data. Mathematica Policy Research has issued a comprehensive report on data quality standards, summarizing the dimensions that should be assessed.[9] Statistics New Zealand has also created a framework for viewing these dimensions that may provide a useful starting point and that may integrate well into federal data strategies.[10] Harron and colleagues (2017) show multiple ways to evaluate linkage across datasets, which are also important when administrative data are not being evaluated on their own.

Data quality issues aside, statistical agencies have a variety of other reasons for investing more heavily in administrative data sources. Administrative data can be used either on their own or in combination with other data. An example of the former is the use of SNAP administrative records to study how SNAP participation increases or declines in response to policy changes. An example of combining administrative data sources is the linking of the Department of Housing and Urban Development's (HUD's) administrative records to SNAP administrative records to estimate the number of households participating in both programs. Administrative data may also be used to enhance the value of survey data or in combination with other administrative data in integrated approaches.

Optimizing the Next Generation Data Platform

A further advantage of administrative data, relative to survey data, is that they exist as a byproduct of routine processes within federal, state, and local governments for such programs as SNAP, WIC, school meals, and others. ERS's Food Economics Division (FED) has improved its capacity to collaborate across agencies using the Next Generation Data Platform (also discussed in detail in Chapter 2) to link administrative data on food assistance programs, survey data, and administrative data on other programs. Through a partnership with the U.S. Census Bureau and sister USDA agency FNS,[11] FED has accessed and analyzed detailed SNAP and WIC data. As of 2017, this partnership included 20 state SNAP agencies (including some counties in California) and 11 state WIC agencies." ERS relies on the Census Bureau's infrastructure to negotiate, ingest, harmonize, and link records. The agency's researchers then access de-identified administrative records that may be linked to survey information (e.g., from the American Community Survey) to assess program eligibility and uptake. The

---

[9]See https://www.mathematica-mpr.com/our-publications-and-findings/publications/transparency-in-the-reporting-of-quality-for-integrated-data-a-review-of-international-standards.

[10]See archive.stats.govt.nz/methods/data.../guide-to-reporting-on-admin-data-quality.aspx.

[11]For information on FNS participation and counts, see https://www.usda.gov/media/blog/2018/01/05/collaboration-across-agencies-supports-food-assistance-research.

success of this partnership relies on the attention and availability of staff, so at times other priorities and projects at the Census Bureau may crowd out this project. ERS should continue its efforts to inventory data available for research use, invest in data documentation, improve data linkage methods, and study the representativeness of Next Generation Data Platform data.

Unfortunately, the usual application process for using the FSRDCs does not give the academic and policy research community easy access to component administrative data and merged administrative and survey data from the Next Generation Data Platform for the SNAP and WIC programs. Existing Census-ERS-FNS data were created with ERS funding, but this was accomplished under the Census Bureau's Census Act authority, so any project using these data must generate a direct benefit to the Census Bureau. This limitation means that some data projects that would be of value specifically to ERS and FED do not qualify, and outside researchers cannot always access these data or know what is available.

In planning for their specific research, policy, and monitoring needs, investment by FED in the Next Generation Data Platform should take into account the planned implementation of the Foundations for Evidence-based Policymaking Act of 2018 (hereafter the Foundations Act), which will require agencies to identify data that can be used to "facilitate the use of evidence in policymaking" and to create for each agency a chief evaluation officer to coordinate evidence-building activities and a chief data officer to oversee "lifecycle data management."[12] Despite the Foundations Act, it is currently unclear when or how federal resources will support the development of a stable, reliable data sharing infrastructure at the federal or state level. The Foundations Act states that "the head of an agency shall, to the extent practicable, make any data asset maintained by the agency available, upon request, to any statistical agency or unit for purposes of developing evidence." This raises the question of which data assets are maintained by FED as part of the CFDS and subject to this new law. Section 3564(f) of the Foundations Act notes that nothing in it preempts applicable state laws regarding the confidentiality of data collected by the states. It is expected that the Office of Management and Budget (OMB) and the statistical agencies will gather, interpret, and deconflict laws and regulations related to data access.

RECOMMENDATION 4.7: To aid ERS in expanding the Next Generation Data platform, intergovernmental coordination is needed to maximize the impacts of infrastructure changes made by the Farm Bill (the Agricultural Improvement Act of 2018) and the Foundations for Evidence-Based Policymaking Act. States and localities should share their administrative data, including SNAP and WIC case records,

[12]This language is contained in the Summary of the Act, which may be found at https://www.congress.gov/bill/115th-congress/house-bill/4174.

with USDA. USDA should optimize use and access through data intermediaries, including but not limited to the Census Bureau. ERS should develop specifications for their process whereby researchers access administrative and commercial data, and for how researcher-provided data can be brought in and linked to other data.

ERS has authority to request information on programs funded by USDA, though ERS has no compelling legislation that forces state and local agencies to share their data. ERS can encourage these agencies to participate in the Next Generation Data Platform by offering technical assistance for data management and analysis or tools that help agencies improve program monitoring and administration.

The Farm Bill states that the Secretary of Agriculture shall provide guidance and direction for interested states on how states should form longitudinal databases supporting research on participation in and the operation of SNAP, including the duration of participation in the program. The Farm Bill further specifies that the guidance will include standard features for the databases, including database formats, data security, and privacy protections; a directive to establish unique identifiers that provide relevant information on household members receiving benefits; direction on funding the establishment and operation of such databases; and a description of the documentation that research users must provide to gain access to the databases. The law advises USDA to consult with states who have built such databases and with the Census Bureau. Implementation guidelines and technical assistance are needed to help states build databases that are interoperable across state lines as well as with other federal program data. One critical factor necessary for promoting state partnerships is to support the development of data documentation and standard schema across existing state and federal administrative sources to improve data harmonization and interoperability.

As described above, the Foundations Act should make data from other agencies available for federal statistical purposes. This could bring information on workforce, housing, justice, and education issues from administrative data into FED studies of program participation. Along these lines, there are other useful models for merging agency data with surveys as well. One example involves linking data on health outcomes from major agencies and programs—including HUD, the SSA, the National Death Index (NDI), and Health and Human Services' (HHS's) Medicare and Medicaid programs—with data from existing surveys conducted by the National Center for Health Statistics. The latter include NHIS, NHANES, the Longitudinal Survey of Aging (LSOA), and others.[13] These types of linked

[13]For information about these data linking efforts, see https://www.cdc.gov/nchs/data-linkage/mortality.htm?CDC_AA_refVal=https%3A%2F%2Fwww.cdc.gov%2Fnchs%2Fdata_access%2Fdata_linkage%2Fmortality.htm.

data have been used, for example, to identify how NHIS parental reports about child asthma correspond to Medicaid data on use of services due to asthma (Zablotsky and Black, 2019). Another example comes from Simon and colleagues (2013). They used linked NHIS-Medicaid data to see what population-level participation by children in Medicaid looks like over a 5-year period, and found that 41 percent of children in the United States were enrolled in Medicaid at some point over 5 years, as compared with 33 percent in a single year.

Numerous administrative sources—such as the Store Tracking and Redemption System (STARS) data on store participation in SNAP and redemptions, and The Integrity Program (TIP) data on WIC store participation, redemptions, and sanctions—are currently reported to FNS but not widely used in research. The same is true of the underlying raw data used to create the SNAP Quality Control datasets and the WIC Participant and Program Characteristics data. It is admirable that some public-use, aggregate versions of these data are available, yet such aggregated data do not contain detail sufficient for some research purposes. Ideally, access to micro versions of WIC Participant and Program Characteristics data, at levels below the state level, would be hosted at ERS or at the FSDRC.

Conclusions about Effective Use of Administrative Data

To fully analyze program participation, eligibility, and take-up through changing social, economic, and policy conditions, administrative data alone are insufficient. Instead, for these purposes administrative data are best used in combination with other kinds of data. Data from surveys and commercial sources can provide more comprehensive information, whether on households or retailers, that can be linked to these administrative data. These sources provide health and nutrition outcome variables that can be used to analyze the effects of participating in programs. They are crucial to analyses of population subgroups, such as veterans, that could not separately be analyzed with administrative data alone. And, by combining administrative data on the use of programs with survey data used to model eligibility, researchers can study take-up patterns and program use among those eligible for the programs. The promise of these types of links can be seen in the two studies using linked NHIS/NHANES-Medicaid data cited above.

For integrating surveys with administrative data, and possibly commercial data, the FED should anticipate data uses in the spirit of small-area estimation. For example, to understand how local labor market conditions affect use of and eligibility for SNAP, researchers need accurate data on participation, income, and other characteristics at the local labor market level to determine eligibility. Similarly, to understand in which communities the SNAP and WIC programs are reaching more eligible people, similar fine geographic data on participation (from administrative sources) and eligibility (derived from survey and possibly administrative data) are needed.

The case for expanded and better coordinated use of administrative data is especially clear for the purposes of program evaluation and improvement, including for SNAP, WIC, school meals, and other program policies. A number of investments will be required to overcome current barriers to the use of administrative data and to make it easier for new states to participate in partnerships with the Census Bureau and for their data to be incorporated.

4.4. OPPORTUNITIES FROM AND CHALLENGES WITH EXPANDING USE OF COMMERCIAL DATA

A forward looking CFDS must anticipate changes in food acquisition among specific groups and be capable of measuring new patterns of food acquisition. This requires thinking about the impacts of emerging food shopping modes such as Amazon and other home food delivery, "grab and go," and the blurring between store-prepared meals and eating at home. In such an environment, the role of data gathered organically in commercial sectors will become increasingly useful for measurement purposes.

The Changing Nature of Commercially Available Data

The past decade has witnessed the emergence of many innovative techniques and approaches that make use of naturally occurring data to measure population characteristics or predict future behavior. The exponential pace of technology change is having a ripple effect on the availability of data in nearly every sector of research and evaluation, including research in the areas of markets, consumer choices and food security, and health and nutrition. This is important, as even the nature of people's behavior and attitudes toward food and purchasing has undergone a radical change. For instance, in some markets there has been a move away from an emphasis on packaged foods, microwavable meals, and shopping the "center aisles" toward an embrace of fresh ingredients, deli-prepared foods, healthier alternatives (e.g., shopping the "edges" where the fresh produce is often located), "grab and go" prepped meals, and transparency of ingredients and calories (Fortson, 2018).

These new sources of data—most often available through commercial research organizations—provide information that can help address critical questions in areas such as (i) diets, nutrition, and obesity; (ii) food security and safety nets; (iii) changing consumer preferences in response to price changes, new information, or product attributes; (iv) the food environment, including the availability of stores and restaurants, food prices in an area, and community characteristics; and (v) industry responses and agricultural sector adaptations to these many changes (Larimore et al., 2018).

It is critical, however, that as these new sources of data become available for use, food researchers and evaluators have a deep and nuanced understanding of the nature of these data and the strengths and weaknesses of each source. Despite their attractive qualities, the value of commercial data can be limited by access issues, coverage and representation bias, lack of documentation or transparency of methods, limited scope of variables, and privacy concerns.

As a general class, such commercial data can be thought of as "organic data" as opposed to "design data" (Groves, 2011). Traditional sources of data—from surveys, censuses, and evaluation studies—often involve a significant design element. That is, the researcher is the one who determines the specific population, how that population is (or is not) to be sampled, the data elements to be collected, and how those data elements will be used in the analysis and to draw insights and conclusions. In short, design data are those over which the researcher has much influence and control.

In contrast, organic data arise out of the broader information ecosystem, that is, they emerge from or are used to drive a process. In this respect, such data are not designed for research purposes, but are more the creation of engineers and computer programmers tasked with running a system or platform; examples include retail UPC scanning systems and an online restaurant or home-food-delivery websites.

These data can have great value in the following ways. First, they tend to be massive. For example, IRI InfoScan provides weekly food purchase data from around 48,000 stores, based on more than 6.6 *billion* observations annually (Levin and Sweitzer, 2018). Second, they provide measurements linked to the events happening in "real time." Retail scanner data, for example, capture the exact time and date of each scanned transaction. Third, they can provide an unobtrusive (or passive) way of measuring phenomena, without the need to directly engage with the subjects of the research or evaluation. For example, store-level retail scanner data are captured as part of the natural store checkout process. However, because these data are not designed or controlled in any way by the researcher, a number of cautions and data evaluation steps should be considered before these data are used (see below for more details).

As noted in a prior National Academies of Sciences, Engineering, and Medicine report (NASEM, 2017a), organic data can vary greatly in their degree of structure, that is, the degree to which data are in a fixed and readily available format for analysis, as contrasted with those data—termed "unstructured data"—which need to undergo some kind of transformation before they can be analyzed (such as images, videos, social media, or

TABLE 4-1 Types of Organic Data by Degree of Structure

	Structured Data–Administrative Records	Other Structured Data	Semi-Structured Data	Unstructured Data
Definition	Data with a fixed format easily exportable to a dataset for analysis with minimal scrubbing required	Highly organized data easily placed in a dataset but requiring additional scrubbing or transformation before analysis	Data that may have some structure (but not complete structure) and cannot be placed in a relational database; require substantial scrubbing	Data that have no standard analytic structure and must have usable data extracted from them and transformed before use
Examples	• Government programs • Commercial transactions • Credit card/bank records • University/school records • Medical records	• e-commerce transactions • Mobile phone GPS	• Computer logs • Text messages • Email • Wearable sensor data • Internet of Things data	• Social media content • Images/videos • Drone data • Satellite/radar information

SOURCE: Adapted (and tailored to food security-related items) from NASEM (2017a).

satellite data). Table 4.1 provides an overview of these categories of data, running from the most to the least structured, as they relate to various sources of potential use in understanding food issues, access, and security. These distinctions are important for differentiating the utility of administrative records versus other types of data that may be commercially available.

Types of Commercial Data, and How They Can Be Used by USDA

Commercial organizations provide an array of structured and unstructured data that are especially useful for improving information about the food environment, such as details about stores and how food is laid out within them; ways of acquiring food; information about prices, quantities, and nutritional values; and other characteristics of individual food items (Burke, 2018). As reviewed in Chapter 2 and summarized in Table 4.2, ERS routinely draws from commercial databases in its ongoing research and evaluation work on consumer food, nutrition, and health. Such data have been used to increase the granularity or timeliness of information and to fill data gaps while, in some cases, also reducing costs and respondent burden.

TABLE 4-2 Commercial Data Sources Routinely Used by ERS

Source	Description
IRI Household	Item-level grocery purchases
IRI Retail	Item-level sales
Nielsen TDLinx	Store characteristics and geocoded location
Nielsen Homescan	Household scanned price and quantity information for package goods
NPD Recount	Restaurant location and characteristics

Sources such as Homescan and retail scanner databases can provide longitudinal measures of consumer choice that, even if imperfect, can be linked to policy or food environment data (Okrent, 2018). These data can provide details about geographic distribution across individual stores or markets, as well as product-level details such as brand, size/weight, and type of package, health and nutrition claims (e.g., gluten-free, type of sugar added, and whether good for reducing risk of heart disease or diabetes). For example, retail scanner data has been linked with nutritional data to create a crosswalk for understanding the relationship between food prices and food purchases (Carlson, 2018). In the near future, such data will also likely provide information about added or supplemental vitamins and minerals, use of non-genetically modified organism (GMO) ingredients or with specialized farming or animal care procedures, and other detailed claims of characteristics about which consumers may care (Burke, 2018). Other potential sources, although not available routinely or systematically, may include data on farmers' markets, food banks, or school lunch suppliers.

ERS is combining IRI InfoScan sales data with sales data from the 2012 and 2017 Economic Census to augment their analytic capacity in a variety of ways. For some chains, IRI only reports sales at the level of the retailers' marketing area so as not to reveal individual store sales, which might help competitors. Yet many uses of interest to ERS require sales to be linked to specific locations. The Economic Census data can be used to help impute disaggregated sales for those stores that report at a metropolitan-area level. Also, many retailers do not report private-label sales (for competitive reasons); nor do they always report random-weight items and perishables, which are important metrics for understanding the food environment. By matching InfoScan stores to stores in the Economic Census, the quality of imputed sales for these items can be improved. Of course, imputations should also be assessed for quality.

Firm-originated data can also be leveraged to evaluate information on food away from home in the IRI Consumer Panel. While the detailed Consumer Panel data are a crucial input for many studies of consumer choice and the food environment, they do not have information on food away from home that is not acquired at food stores. Government survey data can be used to impute information about food consumed away from home to be used in tandem with the Consumer Panel and firm data, again with care to assess the quality of the imputations.

The breadth and depth of commercial data available vary greatly across geographic areas, populations, and programs. Even so, the geospatial aspect of these data can be used, perhaps in tandem with other data, to enable fine geographic assessment of poverty, hunger, and food accessibility (Allard, 2017) and to assess how the food environment can affect consumer choice (Ver Ploeg, Larimore, and Wilde, 2017). For example, NDP Recount provides a near census of data on the locations of food-service operators (both commercial and noncommercial), which can be used to draw insights into (i) restaurant density within a particular area; (ii) the penetration of different types of restaurants within a community; and (iii) comparisons of restaurant revenues across geographies (Hanson and Lesce, 2018). These could also be linked with the other data described above to get a more complete picture of the food environment, to help understand issues related to population changes in an area, or to help understand the impact of the age or racial composition of local neighborhoods. Important features generated from combining the IRI Consumer Panel with data on firms include metrics on the locations of stores used and the distance to the nearest store (accessibility), the assortment of foods sold, the costs required to get to a store, and so on (Bonanno, 2018).

The above examples are suggestive of the potential of commercial data to add new dimensions to ERS's CFDS. It is important that the agency continue its work in this area.

RECOMMENDATION 4.8: The U.S. Department of Agriculture (USDA) should exploit new ideas for integrating commercial data into the Consumer Food Data System. For example, to produce a long "time series" of data on Supplemental Nutrition Assistance Program (SNAP) participation, food insecurity status, and the location of all stores in the immediate environment of the respondent, USDA could facilitate matching restricted-access Food Security Supplement data (with respondents' locations) with TDLinx data on stores, state data on SNAP and other program participation, and Store Tracking and Redemption System data on stores that redeem SNAP.

As commercial data sources are increasingly used to assess food-related issues, a number of priorities for advancing their use have emerged. These include the following:

- Documenting and improving the overall representativeness of retail data.

- Developing weights for the retail stores to make them representative of the geographical areas covered.
- Imputing prices for random weight purchases in the household data.
- Merging prices of products not chosen by consumers as outside options when formally modeling consumer demand systems and choices.
- Imputing prices and/or sales for individual stores and private labels where they have been suppressed and documenting their suppression.
- Linking stores listed in the household Consumer Panel with data generated by those establishments.
- Acquiring new data from vendors, if feasible, on SNAP and WIC variables that are less restricted in use than existing consumer and firm household data.[14]
- Extracting from commercial data sources a variable on the payment method to infer usage of cash, credit, coupons, and SNAP or WIC benefits.

CFDS could productively undertake these project ideas.

Assessing the Quality of Commercial Data

The promise of data beyond surveys and structured administrative data is large, but the benefits are only just beginning to be realized. As with survey and administrative data, commercial data must be evaluated for quality. Like survey and administrative data, these data often suffer from a variety of issues that affect a researcher's ability to truly understand their nature, representativeness, and quality.[15] Also lacking is a set of agreed-upon techniques for assessing the validity, reliability, and robustness of the inferences made from such data. Assessing the quality of data requires a level of transparency. For example, CFDS stewards (and researchers) need to be able to deal with changing platforms among proprietary providers

[14] Current use of the retail data from Nielsen is available for a 5-year window via the Kilts Center for Marketing at the University of Chicago. Data use agreements for these data prevent authors from determining detailed geography, limiting the usefulness of these data. IRI data access via licenses from ERS is limited to users approved by ERS; more open access to these data would increase knowledge. While FNS has data on SNAP redemptions and individual states have data on WIC redemptions of food instruments (in paper-voucher states) and electronic data (in EBT states), these data are used for research only lightly if at all. And these data on redemptions do not inform researchers about what else consumers buy when they are using SNAP or WIC or what they buy on trips when they do not use the vouchers.

[15] See NASEM (2017a, Ch. 4) for a comprehensive discussion of the use of private-sector data for federal statistics.

and to document changes in internal algorithms, an issue especially relevant to proprietary datasets.

RECOMMENDATION 4.9: As with survey and administrative data, commercial data in the Consumer Food Data System should be continually reviewed for accuracy. Data checking, including comparing proprietary commercial data with other sources, such as the Census of Retail Trade, is an essential part of data acquisition, data processing, and vetting. It is important to document coverage of these auxiliary data in terms of geography, the distribution of retail outlets across types, and the amount of purchases captured. It is also important to construct weights to make the population of participants demographically representative of the national population.[16]

Widespread use of commercial data as a replacement for well-designed, representative surveys and more robust and accessible administrative data is still some distance in the future. Nonetheless, ERS has an admirable tradition of using commercial data while also comparing findings, totals, and coverage with other sources.

Given the need to ensure data quality and transparency for research or evaluation purposes, a framework is needed for evaluating potential sources of bias and error. Having such a framework would allow a more systematic and standardized way of assessing datasets before use.

One such framework builds on the concept of Total Survey Error (TSE), which parses potential sources of bias and error broadly into sampling and nonsampling errors (Biemer, 2010). The TSE framework attempts to break down the potential sources of error and variance originating from (a) the sampling process, including errors that occur because only a sample of the population of interest, rather than all of it, is surveyed, and (b) nonsampling components of the survey process, such as frame construction, data collection, data processing and estimation approaches (Biemer, 2010).

A similar yet more expansive framework is needed to assess newer types of nonsurvey data. The outlines of such an approach, which builds on and expands the TSE framework and may be thought of as the Total Data Error (TDE) approach, were described by Japec and colleagues (2015). The TDE framework includes the more traditional sampling error assessments but expands the sources of nonsampling error to include measures of error capturing how commercial or organic data are generated, extracted, transformed, loaded, and ultimately analyzed. The approach attempts to account for a variety of potential errors, such as observation-level errors of omission

[16] Some sources, such as the IRI Consumer Panel, include weights that are provided to ERS as part of the data purchase. Other sources, such as InfoScan data, do not come with weights.

(when relevant cases are excluded due to data selection procedures—similar to survey noncoverage); duplication (depending on how data are captured there may be multiple observations for a single individual or firm); or cases may be included that do not actually match the population of interest).

The potential sources of error extend far beyond those normally encountered in more design-based surveys. As such, it is critical that a framework be developed to help evaluate these potential sources of error in current and future commercial data sources used in food research. Commercial or organic data may have problems related to concept error (when data provided do not actually measure the concept the researcher thinks is being covered) or variability across datasets in the way similar concepts are measured or stored. Likewise, throughout the collection and transformation process, these data may be subject to errors related to how data are extracted, transformed for analyses (particularly in the case of unstructured data), imputed, or analyzed. A TDE framework will account for these newer sources of error to allow for easier and more meaningful assessment of the quality of the data and insights generated from it.

RECOMMENDATION 4.10: The Economic Research Service should develop and use a Total Data Error Framework—which includes the assessment of traditional sampling error and expands on the traditional sources of nonsampling error—to aid in evaluations of the quality and utility of existing and future potential data sources, ranging from commercial or other "organic data" sources to data from surveys and administrative sources. This framework should consider aspects of data origin, generation, extraction, transformation, loading, and analysis in addition to the preceding recommendations for assessing data quality. Standards should be identified and adhered to for gauging the quality of stand-alone data and linkages and to assess privacy risks associated with all components of the Consumer Food Data System.

Data Use and Access

Commercial data are purchased by statistical agencies with the intention that they can be effectively used in a strategy that improves the accuracy or breadth of information, reduces costs or survey burden, or both.

RECOMMENDATION 4.11: The Economic Research Service should continue to invest in efforts to overcome barriers to the use of proprietary data. One element of the strategy should be to negotiate an improvement in terms for Nielsen TDLinx data-sharing agreements to increase the ability to link these data at fine geographic levels and across sources.

Specific examples of the use of such proprietary data include linking the Consumer Panel to the TDLinx data and linking data from either of these sources to detailed Census data on local characteristics or to data on local policies. ERS should act to ensure that other proprietary data also have use terms similarly specified.

Giving researchers access to data is also essential in order to generate value from the investment in it. One challenge with using proprietary commercial data is that access to them is limited. For example, non-ERS-affiliated users can obtain access to retail data from Nielsen through the Kilts Center for Marketing at the University of Chicago's Booth School of Business, but users of these data through Kilts face limits on determining detailed geography. IRI data access via licenses from ERS is limited to ERS-approved users. More open access to these data would increase knowledge.

RECOMMENDATION 4.12: The commercial data in the Consumer Food Data System (CFDS) should also be made more accessible to outside researchers and the policy community while preserving privacy. The U.S. Department of Agriculture should ensure that qualified researchers have access to proprietary data from Nielsen, TDLinx, and other commercial providers in CFDS. Legal barriers—such as indemnity clauses that prevent access to researchers, especially those employed by land-grant and other state-assisted institutions, which are forbidden by state law from entering such agreements—should be eliminated from current and future contracts; or, alternatively, means of data access should be explored while maintaining data privacy and security.

4.5. CREATING COMPREHENSIVE POLICY DATABASES

Policy evaluation should be an important consideration in data collection design. There are important policy questions at each level: program questions at the state level, agency questions at the system level, and outcomes questions at the client level. Often, data belong to the states, and they and local governments administer the policies governing the data's use, but the federal government is paying for some or all of it. Nevertheless, comprehensive databases tracking important policy choices do not exist, and FED faces restrictions on how much and what they ask states, retailers, clinics, and other entities to limit the burden they put on the public.

The SNAP Policy Database and SNAP Distribution Database are model resources for the handling of administrative policy data, allowing research to be carried out about how program choices made by different governmental entities affect outcomes in their localities. These two databases have led to the publication of papers (e.g., Kuhn, 2018; Heflin et al., 2019; Beatty et al., 2019; Ganong and Liebman, 2018) studying the effects of program participation on participant outcomes and on the SNAP cycle.

RECOMMENDATION 4.13: The Supplemental Nutrition Assistance Program (SNAP) Policy Database and the SNAP Distribution Database should be updated annually by the Economic Research Service's (ERS's) Food and Economics Division. Similar cross-state over-time policy databases on additional food assistance programs, such as Special Supplemental Nutrition Program for Women, Infants, and Children (WIC), the School Breakfast Program, the National School Lunch Program, and the Child and Adult Care Food Program should be established and updated annually by ERS. Data that measure rules affecting participating retailers (e.g., stocking requirements) and other entities (e.g., reimbursed foods in school meals programs) should also be collected and made available. Data should be made available about the geographic location of benefit offices (e.g., the city, county, state, latitude, and longitude of locations where participants apply and recertify for assistance, including schools, SNAP offices, and WIC clinics). Finally, administrative data on store participation in SNAP (through the Store Tracking and Redemption System) and WIC (through The Integrity Profile) should be made available with geographic locations for participating retailers; the possibility of making redemption data available should also be explored.

Ideally, data would be included on cash purchases and SNAP or WIC redemptions for the same individuals and sales and redemptions at the same stores so complete acquisitions could be studied.

There have been some successful linkages across survey, administrative, and program-rule databases that have enhanced knowledge. For example, the Census Bureau's American Community Survey has been combined with administrative SNAP records and the SNAP rules database. That linkage is at the household level, which has allowed researchers to answer questions such as, what is the impact of SNAP policy changes on program participation and employment outcomes? This has been successful, but at present easy access is limited to those with internal Census projects, and access only applies to data for the states that participate in the Next Generation Data Platform.

4.6. COMBINING DATA SOURCES AND DATA ACCESS

We conclude with some overarching guidance that applies to more than one aspect of the CFDS as ERS continues to enhance data products through more expansive contracts with proprietary data, states and localities, and links to other federal administrative data. Most critical to this process is continued assessment of the quality of all data, whether survey, commercial, or administrative. Estimates based on different sources should be compared with one another where possible, and the quality of any linkages should be assessed.

Standards are available for gauging the quality of stand-alone data and of linkages and for assessing the privacy risks associated with all components of the CFDS. Some of the sources of these standards operate within the statistical agencies, such as the Federal Committee on Statistical Methodology.[17] Others—such as the Inter-university Consortium for Political and Social Research (ICPSR), a group of more than 750 academic institutions and research organizations that "provides leadership and training in data access, curation, and methods of analysis for the social science research community"[18]—reside outside of government. Elsewhere, a group of researchers at University College London provides guidance for information about linking datasets;[19] and the Harvard Privacy Tools Project seeks to advance "a multidisciplinary understanding of data privacy issues and build computational, statistical, legal, and policy tools to help address these issues in a variety of contexts."[20]

The quality of data can only be thoroughly assessed through regular use of the data by researchers.

RECOMMENDATION 4.14: The Economic Research Service's (ERS's) Food Economics Division should create a process for hosting restricted-use data through a secure platform, such as the Federal Statistical Research Data Centers network. Data for publicly funded programs should be made available for research at granular levels, including individual-level de-identified and linkable data, while still addressing privacy concerns. This should include information generated in activities funded or sponsored by ERS and the Food Nutrition Service, including the food assistance programs and other programs whose output is included in the Consumer Food Data System.

The FSRDC network has a well-established set of enclaves hosting sensitive data. However, costs and conditions for hosting data in the FSRDC are not transparent. Timelines and processes for getting multi-agency projects approved also lack transparency and stability over time, resulting in fragile arrangements often reliant on an agency champion or insistent

---

[17] See https://nces.ed.gov/fcsm.

[18] See https://www.icpsr.umich.edu/icpsrweb.

[19] See https://academic.oup.com/jpubhealth/article/40/1/191/3091693.

[20] See https://privacytools.seas.harvard.edu.

investigator. ERS FED can work on improving conditions in the FSRDC network. FSRDC processes are evolving to streamline requests across many sources of government data (driven in part by the Evidence Act), building upon long-standing processes that supported Census and health agency data access. For example, the FSRDC network has a demonstration project testing secure remote access for approved researchers, potentially aligning the network with other providers who already offer remote research access (e.g., NORC Data Enclave, New York University's Administrative Data Research Facility).

The following issues have been observed in earlier data-sharing efforts and will need to be addressed by ERS FED to increase data access.

1. A broad framework should be created specifying who should get access, including all qualified researchers suitably defined, rather than making data available only to specific subsets of the research community (such as cooperative researchers only, only those with USDA funding, or only for Intergovernmental Personnel Assignment Act reassignments or Schedule A Federal Employees). This will require considering issues like institutional attachment, citizenship, and vetting/background checks. It may also need to vary by researchers' attachment to the government.
2. A broad array of data should be made available at disaggregated but de-identified levels that also contain clear and complete metadata.
3. Costs should be able to be covered by funding from USDA or from external sources (e.g., from reputable federal, state, or nonprofit sources).
4. Automated data provisioning should be used to minimize delays and errors caused by people manually moving files to secure workspaces.
5. Application processes for use of any non-Census Act data at the FSRDCs (via ResearchDataGov) or at an ERS-hosted location should be clearly laid out, following the models of other agencies, such as the Bureau of Labor Statistics, National Center for Health Statistics, and Agency for Healthcare Research and Quality.
6. Best practices for using data collected for other purposes should be delineated.
7. Careful consideration should be given concerning who is allowed to execute linkages of external data. Data-linkage protocols, including use of trusted third parties, should be established.
8. State administrative data used by ERS researchers should follow output review protocols that ensure adherence to project scope and sensitivity while maintaining academic freedom and access to publicly funded data.

9. Proprietary data, such as ERS versions of Nielsen and IRI data, should be housed in such a setting for joint academic research. This may require innovation in the FSRDC network or ERS FED can pursue secure hosting for such data by other service providers.

To ensure that no proprietary, confidential data are being released, FoodAPS requires content and disclosure reviews for projects. Decisions about disclosure should be based on protecting respondents, not based on reviewing the research message—that is, they should be strictly about privacy and confidentiality.

As described throughout this report, analytic capacity can be greatly enhanced when data are combined across a wide range of sources to enable both monitoring and causal research—including scanner data on people and store sales and prices, UPC-level nutrient and product characteristics, food environment data, population-representative survey data, and administrative data on program participation. Taking advantage of multiple data sources requires that the ERS FED partner with other agencies to leverage strengths. For example, ERS may decide it is cost-effective to leverage Census survey methodology expertise for some data projects. In other cases, the agency should take advantage of interagency work on developing standards to assess survey, administrative, and proprietary data.

RECOMMENDATION 4.15: The Economic Research Service's (ERS's) Food Economics Division should create a data council to prioritize which data should be created and specify access rules while ensuring that the Consumer Food Data System addresses ongoing U.S. Department of Agriculture research data needs. This council should also help create and update a longer-term data-infrastructure plan. This plan should balance two goals. Access should be as wide as possible to facilitate policy making, scientific advances, education and training, and public understanding about society. Yet, at the same time, data stewards are ethically and legally obligated to protect privacy and sensitive attributes. ERS should seek input from the American Statistical Association, the federal statistical system, and the broader data and research community on how to prevent re-identification, protect sensitive attributes, and increase access. This data council could also be tasked with setting and reviewing the rules for access to ERS and/or Federal Statistical Research Data Centers, described above. This approach could follow the model of the Department of Health and Human Services' data council, and it should include nongovernment stakeholders.

Finally, the CFDS will need to remain open to future changes in how people in the United States acquire and prepare food, what they eat, and how it affects health. This will require paying attention to changing demographics—for example, an aging society may require more congregate meals. Moreover, climate change may lead to changes in how food is produced and what it costs, and changes in technology are sure to affect what food is available.

We have made a series of recommendations that span the current and past CFDS and also make suggestions for the future. Listed here are those that we regard as the highest priority relative to the rest (but not in priority order): (1) recommendations related to checking data and linkage quality, (2) recommendations to enhance more access to existing data and future data by outside researchers as well as through existing relationships with more geography, (3) recommendations laying out strategies to include more administrative data into the CFDS, (4) recommendations that the CFDS systematically focus on serving monitoring needs (e.g., measuring food security consistently) and causal research needs through longitudinal designs, and (5) recommendations to create policy data bases to enhance causal research.

References

Allard, S.W. (2017). *Places in Need: The Changing Geography of Poverty.* New York: Russell Sage Foundation.

Allcott, H., Diamond, R., Jean-Pierre Dube, J., Handbury, J., Rahkovsky, I., and Schnell, M. (2019). Food deserts and the causes of nutritional inequality. *The Quarterly Journal of Economics, 134*(4), 1793–1844.

Anekwe, T.D., and Zeballos, E. (2019). *Food-Related Time Use: Changes and Demographic Differences.* Economic Research Service Economic Information Bulletin No. 213 (Nov.). Available: https://www.ers.usda.gov/webdocs/publications/95399/eib-213.pdf?v=8128.7.

Arteaga, I., and Heflin, C. (2014). Participation in the National School Lunch Program and food security: An analysis of transitions into kindergarten. *Children and Youth Services Review, 47*(P3), 224–230.

Basu, S., Berkowitz, S.A. and Seligman, H. (2017). The monthly cycle of hypoglycemia: an observational claims-based study of emergency room visits, hospital admissions, and costs in a commercially insured population. *Medical Care, 55*(7):639–645

Basu, S., Wimer, C., and Seligman, H. (2016). Moderation of the relation of county-level cost of living to nutrition by the supplemental nutrition assistance program. *American Journal of Public Health, 106*(11), 2064–2070.

Beatty, T.K.M., and Tuttle, C.J. (2015). Expenditure response to increases in in-kind transfers: Evidence from the Supplemental Nutrition Assistance Program. *American Journal of Agricultural Economics, 97*(2), 390–404.

Beatty, T.K.M., Bitler, M., Cheng, X.H., and van der Werf, C. (2019). SNAP and paycheck cycles. *Southern Economic Journal, 86*(1), 18–48.

Benjamin, E.J., Blaha, M.J., Chiuve, S.E., Cushman, M., Das, S.R., Deo, R., de Ferranti, S.D., Floyd, J., Fornage, M., et al. (2017). Heart disease and stroke statistics: 2017 update. A report from the American Heart Association. *Circulation, 135*(10), 135–146.

Bhattacharya, J., Currie, J., and Haider, S. (2004). Poverty, food insecurity, and nutritional outcomes in children and adults. *Journal of Health Economics, 23*, 839–862.

Biemer, P.B. (2010). Total survey error: Design, implementation, and evaluation. *Public Opinion Quarterly 74*, 817–848.

Biemer, P.B., and Amaya, A. (2018). *A Total Error Framework for Hybrid Estimation*. Paper presented at the BigSurv18 Conference, Oct. 26, Barcelona, Spain.

Bollinger, C.R., Hirsch, B., Hokayem, C., and Ziliak, J.P. (2019). Trouble in the tails? What we know about earnings nonresponse thirty years after Lillard, Smith, and Welch. *Journal of Political Economy*. https://doi.org/10.1086/701807.

Bonanno, A. (2018). *Improving Geospatial Information in ERS's Food Data System (Assessing the Role of Accessibility of Food Outlets Role in SNAP Participation and Effectiveness)*. Presentation to the Committee on National Statistics' Panel on Improving USDA's Consumer Data for Food and Nutrition Policy Research, Sept. 21, Washington DC.

Bronchetti, E., Christensen, G., and Hoynes, H. (2019). Local food prices, SNAP purchasing power, and child health, *Journal of Health Economics, 68*(Dec.). https://doi.org/10.1016/j.jhealeco.2019.10223.

Burke, B. (2018). *Leveraging Big Data to Drive Big Growth*. Presentation to the Committee on National Statistics' Panel on Improving USDA's Consumer Data for Food and Nutrition Policy Research, June 14, Washington DC.

Capps, R.W., Gelatt, J.M., and Fix, M. (2018). Commentary on "The number of undocumented immigrants in the United States: Estimates based on demographic modeling with data from 1990–2016." *PLOS One*. https://doi.org10.1371/journal.pone.0204199.

Carlson, A.C. (2018). *Linking Scanner Data to Nutrition Data*. Presentation to the Committee on National Statistics' Panel on Improving USDA's Consumer Data for Food and Nutrition Policy Research, April 16, Washington DC.

Carlson, A.C., Page, E.T., Zimmerman, T.P., Tornow, C.E., and Hermansen, S. (2019). *Linking USDA Nutrition Databases to IRI Household-based and Store-based Scanner Data*. Economic Research Service Technical Bulletin No.1952 (March). Available: https://www.ers.usda.gov/webdocs/publications/92571/tb-1952.pdf?v=8814.2.

Centers for Medicare & Medicaid Services. (2017). *NHE Fact Sheet*. Baltimore, MD.

Chang, Y., Kim, J., and Chatterjee, S. (2017). The association between consumer competency and Supplemental Nutrition Assistance Program participation on food insecurity. *Journal of Nutrition Education and Behavior, 49*(8), 657–666.

Commission on Evidence-Based Policymaking. (2017). *The Promise of Evidence-Based Policymaking: Report of the Commission on Evidence-Based Policymaking*. Washington, DC. Available: https://www.cep.gov/content/dam/cep/report/cep-final-report.pdf.

Courtemanche, C., Denteh, A., and Tchernis, R. (2019). Estimating the associations between SNAP and food insecurity, obesity, and food purchases with imperfect administrative measures of participation. *Southern Economic Journal, 86*(1), 202–228.

Cuffey, J., and Beatty, T. (2019). *Consumer Choice of Store Format: Response to Policy*. Available: https://conservancy.umn.edu/bitstream/handle/11299/200209/Cuffey_umn_0130E_19511.pdf?sequence=1&isAllowed=y.

Denbaly, M. (2018). *Consumer and Food Industry Data System*. Presentation to Committee on National Statistics' Panel on Improving USDA's Consumer Data for Food and Nutrition Policy Research, April 16, Washington DC.

Deshpande, M., and Li, Y. (June 2017). *Who Is Screened Out? Application Costs and the Targeting of Disability Programs*. NBER Working Paper No. 23472. Cambridge, MA: National Bureau of Economic Research.

Dong, D., Stewart, H., Frazão, E., Carlson, A., and Hyman, J. (2016, May). *WIC Household Food Purchases Using WIC Benefits or Paying Out of Pocket: A Case Study of Cold Cereal Purchases*. ERR-207. Washington, DC: U.S. Department of Agriculture, Economic Research Service. Available: https://www.ers.usda.gov/publications/pub-details/?pubid=45536.

Dorfman, J.H., Gregory, C., Liu, Z., and Huo, R. (2018). Re-examining the SNAP benefit cycle allowing for heterogeneity. *Applied Economic Perspectives and Policy 41*(3), 404–433.

Downing, J., and Laraia, B. (2016). *Supermarket Proximity and Price: Food Insecurity and Obesity in the United States*. Lexington: University of Kentucky Center for Poverty Research. Available: https://uknowledge.uky.edu/ukcpr_papers/117.

Duffey, K.J., Gordon-Larsen, P., Shikany, J.M., Guilkey, D., Jacobs, D.R., and Popkin, B.M. (2010). Food price and diet and health outcomes: 20 years of the CARDIA Study. *Archives of Internal Medicine 170*(5), 420–426.

Duncan, G.J., and Kalton, G. (1987). Issues of design and analysis of surveys across time. *International Statistical Review*, (1), 97–117. Available: http://www.jstor.org/stable/1403273.

Einav, L., Leibtag, E., and Nevo, A. (2008). *On the Accuracy of Nielsen Homescan Data*. ERS No. 69. Washington, DC: U.S. Department of Agriculture, Economic Research Service. Available: https://www.ers.usda.gov/publications/pub-details/?pubid=46114.

Einav, L., Leibtag, E., and Nevo, A. (2010). Recording discrepancies in Nielsen Homescan data: Are they present and do they matter? *Quantitative Marketing and Economics, 8*(2), 207–239.

Eltinge, J. (2018). *Inferential Quality and Data Quality in the Integration of Multiple Data Sources*. Presentation to Committee on National Statistics' Panel on Improving USDA's Consumer Data for Food and Nutrition Policy Research, Sept. 21, Washington, DC.

Fang, D., Thomsen, M.R., Nayga, R.M., and Novotny, A.M. (2019). WIC participation and relative quality of household food purchases: Evidence from FoodAPS. *Southern Economic Journal*, 86(1), 83–105.

Feeding America. (2019). *Map the Meal Gap*. Chicago, IL. Available: https://www.feedingamerica.org/sites/default/files/2019-05/2017-map-the-meal-gap-full.pdf.

Finkelstein, A., and Notowidigdo, M.J. (2019). Take-up and targeting: Experimental evidence from SNAP. *The Quarterly Journal of Economics, 134*(3), 1505–1556.

Fortson, J. (2018). *Challenges in Changing Consumer Landscape*. Presentation to Committee on National Statistics' Panel on Improving USDA's Consumer Data for Food and Nutrition Policy Research, June 14, Washington DC.

Frisvold, D., and Price, J. (2019). The contribution of the school environment to the overall food environment experienced by children. *Southern Economic Journal, 86*(1), 106–123.

Ganong, P., and Liebman, J.B. (2018). The decline, rebound, and further rise in SNAP enrollment: Disentangling business cycle fluctuations and policy changes. *American Economic Journal: Economic Policy, 10*(4)153–176.

Giombi, K., Muth, M., and Levin, D. (2018). A comparative analysis of hedonic models of nutrition information and health claims on food products: An application to soup products. *Journal of Food Products Marketing, 24*(1), 1–21.

Gorski, M., and Roberto, C. (2015). Public health policies to encourage healthy eating habits: Recent perspectives. *Journal of Healthcare Leadership 7*, 81–90. https://doi.org/10.2147/JHL.S69188.

Gregory, C.A., and Coleman-Jensen, A. (2013). Do high food prices increase food insecurity in the United States? *Applied Economic Perspectives and Policy, 35*(4), 679–707. https://academic.oup.com/aepp/article/35/4/679/8547/Do-High-Food-Prices-Increase-Food-Insecurity-in.

Gregory, C.A., and Smith, T.A. (2019). Salience, food security, and SNAP receipt. *Journal of Policy Analysis and Management, 38*(1), 124–154.

Groves, R.M. (2011). *Census Directors Blog: Designed Data and Organic Data*. Available: https://www.census.gov/newsroom/blogs/director/2011/05/designed-data-and-organic-data.html.

Groves, R.M., Fowler, F.J., Jr., Couper, M.P., Lepkowski, J.M., Singer, E., and Tourangeau, R. (2009). *Survey Methodology* (2nd ed.). New York: John Wiley and Sons.

Gundersen, C., and Ribar, D.C. (2011). Food insecurity and insufficiency at low levels of food expenditures. *Review of Income and Wealth, 57*(4), 704–726. https://doi.org/10.1111/j.1475-4991.2011.00471.x.

Gundersen, C., and Ziliak, J.P. (2008). The age gradient in Food Stamp Program participation: Does income volatility matter? In D. Jolliffe and J. Ziliak (eds.), *Income Volatility and Food Assistance in the United States* (pp. 171–216). Kalamazoo, MI: W.E. Upjohn Institute for Employment Research.

Gundersen, C., and Ziliak, J.P. (2018, March). Food insecurity research in the United States: Where we have been and where we need to go. *Applied Economic Perspectives and Policy, 40*(1), 119–135. https//doi.org/10.1093/aepp/ppx058.

Gundersen, C., Kreider, B., and Pepper, J. (2017). Partial identification methods for evaluating food assistance programs: A case study of the causal impact of SNAP on food insecurity. *American Journal of Agricultural Economics, 99*(4), 875–894.

Hamilton, W.L., Cook, J.T., Thompson, W.W., Buron, L.F., Frongillo, E.A., Olson, C.M., and Wehler, C.A. (1997). *Household Food Security in the United States in 1995: Technical Report of the Food Security Measurement Project.* Report prepared for USDA Food and Consumer Service. Cambridge, MA: Abt Associates, Inc. Available: http://citeseerx.ist.psu.edu/viewdoc/download;jsessionid=BAB83524BFE1C9351EADA91580281878?doi=10.1.1.26.1356&rep=rep1&type=pdf.

Hanson, A., and Lesce, L. (2018). *NDP's Food Industry Information.* Presentation to Committee on National Statistics' Panel on Improving USDA's Consumer Data for Food and Nutrition Policy Research, June 14, Washington DC.

Harron, K.L., Doidge, J.C., Knight, H.E., Gilbert, R.E. Goldstein, H. Cromwell, D.A., and van der Meulen, J.H. (2017). A guide to evaluating linkage quality for the analysis of linked data. *International Journal of Epidemiology, 46*(5), 1699–1710. https//doi.org/10.1093/ije/dyx177.

Hastings, J., and Shapiro, J.M. (2018). How are SNAP benefits spent? Evidence from a retail panel. *American Economic Review, 108*(12), 3493–3540. https://doi.org/10.1257/aer.20170866.

Heflin, C.M., Ingram, S.J., and Ziliak, J.P. (2019). The effect of the Supplemental Nutrition Assistance Program on mortality. *Health Affairs, 38*(11), 1807–1815.

Hernán M.A., Alonso A., Logan R., Grodstein F., Michels K.B., Willett W.C., Manson J.E., and Robins, J.M. (2008). Observational studies analyzed like randomized experiments: An application to postmenopausal hormone therapy and coronary heart disease (with discussion). *Epidemiology, 19*(6), 766–779.

Hillier, A., Smith, T.E., Whiteman, E.D., and Chrisinger, B.W. (2017). Discrete choice model of food store trips using National Household Food Acquisition and Purchase Survey (FoodAPS). *International Journal of Environmental Research and Public Health, 14*(10), 1133.

Hogue, C., and Dumbacher, B. (2018). *Modernizing Census Bureau Economic Statistics Through Web Scraping and Other Non-Survey Data Sources.* Presentation to Committee on National Statistics' Panel on Improving USDA's Consumer Data for Food and Nutrition Policy Research, Sept. 21, Washington DC.

Hoynes, H.W., and Schanzenbach, D.W. (2015). *U.S. Food and Nutrition Programs.* NBER Working Paper 21057. Cambridge, MA: National Bureau of Economic Research. Available: https://www.nber.org/papers/w21057.

Hu, M., Gremel, G.W., Kirlin, J.A., and West, B.T. (2018). Nonresponse and underreporting errors increase over the data collection week based on paradata from the National Household Food Acquisition and Purchase Survey. *The Journal of Nutrition, 147*(5), 964–975.

Japec, L., Kreuter, F. Berg, M., Biemer, P., Decker, P., Lampe, C., Lane, J., O'Neil, C., and Usher, A. (2015). Big data in survey research: AAPOR Task Force report. *Public Opinion Quarterly, 79*, 839–880.

Jensen, H. (2018). *Understanding WIC Data: Issues with Proprietary (Scanner) Data.* Presentation to Committee on National Statistics' Panel on Improving USDA's Consumer Data for Food and Nutrition Policy Research, Sept. 21, Washington, DC.

Jo, Y. (2017). *The Differences in Characteristics Among Households With and Without Obese Children: Findings from USDA's FoodAPS.* Economic Research Service Economic Information Bulletin No. 179 (Sept.). Available: https://www.ers.usda.gov/publications/pub-details/?pubid=85027.

Kabbani, N., and Wilde, P. (2003). Short recertification periods in the U.S. Food Stamp Program. *The Journal of Human Resources, 38*(Special Issue on Income Volatility and Implications for Food Assistance Programs), 1112–1138.

Kang, K., and Moffitt, R. (2019). The effect of SNAP and school food programs on food security, diet quality, and food spending: Sensitivity to program reporting error. *Southern Economic Journal, 86*(1), 156–253.

Kirlin, J.A., and Denbaly, M. (2017). Lessons learned from the national household food acquisition and purchase survey in the United States, *Food Policy, 72*(October), 62–71.

Krenzke T., and Kali, J. (2016). *Review of the FoodAPS 2012 Sample Design.* Prepared for the Economic Research Service, U.S. Department of Agriculture, Washington, DC.

Kuhn, M.A. (2018). Who feels the calorie crunch and when? The impact of school meals on cyclical food insecurity. *Journal of Public Economics, 166,* 27–38.

Larimore, E., Prell, M., Sweitzer, M., and Variyam, J. (2018). *Improving the Consumer Food Data System.* White Paper. Administrative Publication by the Economic Research Service.

Lazer, D., Kennedy, R., King, G., and Vespignani, A. (2014). The parable of Google flu: Traps in big data analysis. *Science, 343,* 1203–1205.

Leibtag, E., and Kaufman, P. (2003). *Exploring Food Purchase Behavior of Low-Income Households: How Do They Economize?* Economic Research Service Agricultural Information Bulletin 747-07. Available: https://pdfs.semanticscholar.org/5727/c0fd24c7944f835ce562ef4c57060e93d065.pdf.

Levin, D., and Sweitzer, M. (2018). *Use of Proprietary Data.* Presentation to Committee on National Statistics' Panel on Improving USDA's Consumer Data for Food and Nutrition Policy Research, April 16, Washington, DC.

Levin, D., Noriega, D., Dicken, C., Okrent, A., Harding, M., and Lovenheim, M. (2018). *Examining Store Scanner Data: A Comparison of the IRI Infoscan Data with Other Data Sets, 2008-12.* Economic Research Service Technical Bulletin 1949. Available: https://www.ers.usda.gov/publications/pub-details/?pubid=90354.

Lusk, J., and Brooks, K. (2011). Who participates in household scanning panels? *American Journal of Agricultural Economics, 93*(1), 226–240. Available: http://www.jstor.org/stable/41240270.

Mabli, J., and Ohls, J. (2012). Supplemental Nutrition Assistance Program dynamics and employment transitions: The role of employment instability. *Applied Economic Perspectives and Policy, 34*(1), 187–213.

Maitland, A., and Li, L. (2016). *Review of the Completeness and Accuracy of FoodAPS 2012 Data.* Prepared for the Economic Research Service, U.S. Department of Agriculture.

Mancino, L., Guthrie, J., Ver Ploeg, M., and Lin, B (2018). *Nutritional Quality of Foods Acquired by Americans: Findings from USDA's National Household Food Acquisition and Purchase Survey.* Available: https://www.ers.usda.gov/webdocs/publications/87531/eib-188.pdf?%20v=43151.

Marshall, M., Burrows, T., and Collins, C.E. (2014). Systematic review of diet quality indices and their associations with health-related outcomes in children and adolescents. *Journal of Human Nutrition and Dietetics 27,* 577–598.

Meyer, B.D., and N. Mittag, N. (2019). Misreporting of government transfers: How important are survey design and geography? *Southern Economic Journal, 86*(1), 230–253.

Meyer, B.D., Mittag, N., and Goerge, R.M. (2018). *Errors in Survey Reporting and Imputation and their Effects on Estimates of Food Stamp Program Participation.* NBER Working Paper No. 25143. Cambridge, MA: National Bureau of Economic Research. Available: https://www.nber.org/papers/w25143.

Meyer, B.D., Mok, W.K.C., and Sullivan, J.X. (2015). *Household Surveys in Crisis.* NBER Working Paper 21399. Cambridge, MA: National Bureau of Economic Research Available: http://www.nber.org/papers/w21399.

Milken Institute. (2016). *Weighing Down America: The Health and Economic Impact of Obesity.* H. Waters and R. DeVol (eds). Available: https://milkeninstitute.org/reports/weighing-down-america-health-and-economic-impact-obesity.

Miller, D. P., and Morrissey, T. (2017). *Using Natural Experiments to Identify the Effects of SNAP on Child and Adult Health.* University of Kentucky Center for Poverty Research Discussion Paper Series, DP2017-04. Available: https://uknowledge.uky.edu/ukcpr_papers/105.

Mills, G., Vericker, T., Koball, H., Lippold, K., Wheaton, L., and Elkin, S. (2014). *Understanding the Rates, Causes, and Costs of Churning in the Supplemental Nutrition Assistance Program (SNAP).* Washington, DC: U.S. Department of Agriculture, Food and Nutrition Service, Office of Policy Support.

Muth, M.K. (2018). *Store and Household Scanner Data for Food and Nutrition Policy Research.* Presentation to Committee on National Statistics' Panel on Improving USDA's Consumer Data for Food and Nutrition Policy Research, Sept. 21, Washington, DC.

Muth, M.K., Bradley, S.R., Brophy, J.E., Capogrossi, K.L., Coglaiti, M.C., and Karns, S.A. (2015, June). *2014 FDA Labeling Cost Model.* Prepared for U.S. Food and Drug Administration. Research Triangle Park, NC: RTI International. Available: https://www.rti.org/publication/2014-fda-labeling-cost-model

Muth, M.K., Cates, S.C., Karns, S.A., Siegel, P.H., Wohlgenant, K.C., and Zhen, C. (2013, March). *Comparing Attitudinal Survey Responses from Proprietary and Government Surveys.* Prepared for U.S. Department of Agriculture, Economic Research Service.

Muth, M.K., Karns, S.A., Nielsen, S.J., Buzby, J.C., and Wells, H.F. (2011). *Consumer-level Food Loss Estimates and Their Use in the ERS Loss-adjusted Food Availability Data.* Technical Bulletin No. 1927. Available: https://www.ers.usda.gov/webdocs/publications/47570/8043_tb1927.pdf?v=0.

Muth, M.K., Siegel, P.H., and Zhen, C. (2007, February). *ERS Data Quality Study Design.* Prepared for U.S. Department of Agriculture, Economic Research Service. Research Triangle Park, NC: RTI International.

Muth, M.K., Sweitzer, M., Brown, D., Capogrossi, K., Karns, S., Levin, D., Okrent, A., Siegel, P., and Zhen, C. (2016). *Understanding IRI Household-Based and Store-Based Scanner* Data, TB-1942. Washington, DC: U.S. Department of Agriculture, Economic Research Service. Available: https://www.ers.usda.gov/publications/pub-details/?pubid=47636.

NASEM (National Academies of Sciences, Engineering, and Medicine). (2017a). *Innovations in Federal Statistics: Combining Data Sources While Protecting Privacy.* Washington, DC: The National Academies Press. https://doi.org/10.17226/24652.

NASEM. (2017b). *Review of WIC Food Packages: Improving Balance and Choice: Final Report.* Washington, DC: The National Academies Press. https://doi.org/10.17226/23655.

NRC (National Research Council). (1984). *National Survey Data on Food Consumption: Uses and Recommendations.* Washington, DC: The National Academy Press. https://doi.org/10.17226/733.

______. (2005). *Improving Data to Analyze Food and Nutrition Policies.* Panel on Enhancing the Data Infrastructure in Support of Food and Nutrition Programs, Research, and Decision Making, Committee on National Statistics, Division of Behavioral and Social Sciences and Education. Washington, DC: The National Academies Press.

______. (2006). *Food Insecurity and Hunger in the United States: An Assessment of the Measure.* Panel to Review the U.S. Department of Agriculture's Measurement of Food Insecurity and Hunger (G.S. Wunderlich and J.L. Norwood, eds.), Committee on National Statistics, Division of Behavioral and Social Sciences and Education. Washington, DC: The National Academies Press.

NRC and IOM (Institute of Medicine). (2013). *Research Opportunities Concerning the Causes and Consequences of Food Insecurity and Hunger: A Workshop Summary.* N. Kirkendall, C. House, and C.F. Citro, rapporteurs. Committee on National Statistics, Division of Behavioral and Social Sciences and Education. Food and Nutrition Board, Institute of Medicine. Washington, DC: The National Academies Press.

Newman, C., and Scherpf, E. (2013). *Supplemental Nutrition Assistance Program (SNAP) Access at the State and County Levels: Evidence from Texas SNAP Administrative Records and the American Community Survey.* Economic Research Report No. 156. Available: https://www.ers.usda.gov/publications/pub-details/?pubid=45139.

Okrent, A. (2018). *The Strengths and Weaknesses of Using Proprietary Data for Food Policy Analysis.* Presentation to Committee on National Statistics' Panel on Improving USDA's Consumer Data for Food and Nutrition Policy Research, June 14, Washington, DC.

Oliveira, V. (2017). *The Food Assistance Landscape: FY 2016 Annual Report.* EIB 169. Washington, DC: U.S. Department of Agriculture, Economic Research Service. Available: https://www.ers.usda.gov/publications/pub-details/?pubid=82993.

Oliveira, V. (2018). *The Food Assistance Landscape: FY2017 Annual Report.* EIB-190. Washington, DC: U.S. Department of Agriculture, Economic Research Service.

Olson, C.M. (1999). Nutrition and health outcomes associated with food insecurity and hunger. *The Journal of Nutrition 129*(2), 521S–524S. https://doi.org/10.1093/jn/129.2.521S.

Page, E.T., Larimore, E., Kirlin, J.A., and Denbaly, M. (2019). The National Household Food Acquisition and Purchase Survey: Innovations and research insights. *Applied Economic Perspectives and Policy, 41*(2), 215–234. https://doi.org/10.1093/aepp/ppy034.

Petraglia, E., Van de Kerckhove, W., and Krenzke, T. (2016). *Review of the Potential for Nonresponse Bias in FoodAPS 2012.* Prepared for the Economic Research Service, U.S. Department of Agriculture, Washington, DC.

Poti, J, Yoon, E., Hollingsworth, B., Ostrowski, J., Wandell, J., Miles, D, and Popkin, B. (2017). Development of a food composition database to monitor changes in packaged foods and beverage. *Journal of Food Composition and Analysis, 64*(pt. 1), 18–26.

Prell, M. (2016). *llluminating SNAP Performance Using the Power of Administrative Data.* Available: https://www.ers.usda.gov/amber-waves/2016/november/illuminating-snap-performance-using-the-power-of-administrative.

Prell, M. (2018). *Collaboration across Agencies Supports Food Assistance Research.* Available: https://www.usda.gov/media/blog/2018/01/05/collaboration-across-agencies-supports-food-assistance-research.

Rastogi, S., O'Hara, A., Noon, J., Zapata, E.A., Espinoza, C., Marshall, L.B., Schellhamer, T.A., and Brown, J.D. (2010). *Census Match Study.* Center for Administrative Records Research and Applications Report. Washington, DC: U.S. Census Bureau.

Restepro, B., Minor, T., and Peckham, J. (2018). *The Association Between Restaurant Menus Label Use and Caloric Intake.* Economic Research Service Report Number 259. Available: https://www.ers.usda.gov/webdocs/publications/90498/err-259.pdf?v=7741.5.

Restrepo, B., and Zeballos, E. (2019). Time spent eating varies by age, education and body mass index. *Amber Waves*, April 1. Available: https://www.ers.usda.gov/publications/?topicid=14833#!topicid=&subtopicid=&series=&authorid=0&page=4&sortfield=date&sortascending=false.

Rhone, A., ver Ploeg, M., Dicken, C., Williams, R., and Breneman, V. (2017). *Low-Income and Low-Supermarket-Access Census Tracts, 2010-2015*. EIB-165. Available: https://www.ers.usda.gov/publications/pub-details/?pubid=82100.

Ribar, D.C., and Edelhoch, M. (2008). Earnings volatility and the reasons for leaving the food stamp program. In D. Jolliffe and J.P. Ziliac (eds.), *Income Volatility and Food Assistance in the United States* (pp. 63-102). Kalamazoo, MI: W.E. Upjohn Institute.

Ribar, D., and C.A. Swann. (2014). If at first you don't succeed: Applying for and staying on the Supplemental Nutrition Assistance Program. *Applied Economics 46*(27), 3339–3350.

Rigdon, J., Berkowitz, Seligman, H.K., and Basu, S. (2017). Re-evaluating associations between the Supplemental Nutrition Assistance Program participation and body mass index in the context of unmeasured confounders. *Social Science and Medicine, 192*, 112–124.

Scherpf, E., Newman, C., and Prell, M. (2015). *Improving the Assessment of SNAP Targeting Using Administrative Records*. Available: https://ideas.repec.org/p/ags/uersrr/206417.html.

Schmidt, L., Shore-Sheppard, L., and Watson, T. (2016). The effect of safety-net programs on food insecurity. *Journal of Human Resources, 51*(3)589–614.

Shapiro, J. (2005). Is there a daily discount rate? Evidence from the Food Stamp Nutrition Cycle. *Journal of Public Economics, 89*(2–3).

Simon, A.E., Driscoll, A., Gorina, Y., Parker, J.D, and Schoendorf, K.C. (2013). A longitudinal view of child enrollment in Medicaid. *Pediatrics, 132*(4), 656–662.

Smith, T., Berning, J., Yang, X., Colson, G., and Dorfman, J. (2016). The effects of benefit timing and income fungibility on food purchasing decisions among Supplemental Nutrition Assistance Program households. *American Journal of Agricultural Economics, 98*(2), 564–580. https://doi.org/10.1093/ajae/aav072.

Stewart, H., Hyman, J., Carlson, A., and Frazão, E. (2016). *The Cost of Satisfying Fruit and Vegetable Recommendations in the Dietary Guidelines*. EB-27. Washington, DC: U.S. Department of Agriculture, Economic Research Service. https://www.ers.usda.gov/publications/pub-details/?pubid=42904.

Swann, C.A. (2017). Household history, SNAP participation, and food insecurity. *Food Policy*, *73*(C), 1–9.

Sweitzer, M., Brown, D., Karns, S., Muth, M.K., Siegel, P., and Zhen, C. (2018). *Food-at-Home Expenditures: Comparing Commercial Household Scanner Data from IRI and Government Survey Data*. TB-1946. Available: https://www.ers.usda.gov/publications/pub-details/?pubid=85251.

Taylor, R.L., and Villas-Boas, S.B. (2016a). Food store choices of poor households: A discrete choice analysis of the National Household Food Acquisition and Purchase Survey (FoodAPS). *American Journal of Agricultural Economics, 98*(4), 513–532.

Taylor, R.L., and Villas-Boas, S.B. (2016b). Store choice among low-income households. *American Journal of Agricultural Economics 98*(2), 513–532. doi: 10.1093/ajae/aaw009.

Tiehen, L., Newman, C., and Kirlin, J. (2017). *The Food-Spending Patterns of Households Participating in the Supplemental Nutrition Assistance Program: Findings from USDA's FoodAPS*. EIB 176. Available: https://www.ers.usda.gov/publications/pub-details?pubid=84779.

Todd, J., and Scharadin, B. (2016). *Where Households Get Food in a Typical Week: Findings from USDA's FoodAPS*. EIB-156. Available: https://www.ers.usda.gov/publications/pub-details/?pubid=80541.

Todd, J., Leibtag, E., and Penberthy, C. (2011). *Geographic Differences in the Relative Price of Healthy Foods*, EIB-78. Available: https://www.ers.usda.gov/publications/pub-details/?pubid=44562.

U.S. Departments of Agriculture and Health and Human Services. (2015). *Scientific Report of the 2015 Dietary Guidelines Advisory Committee, Part. D. Chapter 4*. Available: https://health.gov/dietaryguidelines/2015-scientific-report.

U.S. Office of Management and Budget. (2005). *Policy Working Paper 22. Report on Statistical Disclosure Limitation Methodology.* Available: https://www.hhs.gov/sites/default/files/spwp22.pdf.

U.S. Office of Management and Budget. (2014). *M-14-06: Guidance for Providing and Using Administrative Data for Statistical Purposes.* Available: https://obamawhitehouse.archives.gov/sites/default/files/omb/memoranda/2014/m-14-06.pdf.

U.S. Office of Management and Budget. (2016). Building the capacity to produce and use evidence. In *Analytical Perspectives: Budget of the United States Government: Fiscal Year 2017* (Ch. 7, pp. 69–77). Available: https://obamawhitehouse.archives.gov/sites/default/files/omb/budget/fy2017/assets/ap_7_evidence.pdf.

Ver Ploeg, M., Larimore, E., and Wilde, P. (2017). *The Influence of Food Store Access on Grocery Shopping and Food Spending.* EIB-180. Available: https://www.ers.usda.gov/publications/pub-details/?pubid=85441.

Ver Ploeg, M., Mancino, L., Todd, J.E. Clay, D.M., and Scharadin, B. (2015). *Where Do Americans Usually Shop for Food and How Do They Travel to Get There? Initial Findings from the National Household Food Acquisition and Purchase Survey.* EIB-138. Available: https://www.ers.usda.gov/publications/pub-details/?pubid=79791.

Ver Ploeg, M. (2018). *Linking to Food Environment Data.* Presentation to the Committee on National Statistics' Panel on Improving USDA's Consumer Data for Food and Nutrition Policy Research, April 16, Washington, DC.

Wendt, M., and Todd, J. (2011). *The Effect of Food and Beverage Prices on Children's Weights.* ERR-118. Available: https://www.ers.usda.gov/publications/pub-details/?pubid=44851.

Whiteman, E.D., Chrisinger, B.W., and Hillie, A. (2018). Diet quality over the monthly Supplemental Nutrition Assistance Program cycle. *American Journal of Preventive Medicine, 55*(2), 2105–2012.

Wilde, P. (2004). *The Uses and Purposes of the USDA Food Security and Hunger Measure: A Report for the Committee on National Statistics Panel on Food Security Measurement.* Tufts University Friedman School of Nutrition Science and Policy.

Wilde, P., and Ismail, M. (2018). *Review of the National Household Food Acquisition and Purchase Survey (FoodAps) from a Data User's Perspective.* Available: https://www.ers.usda.gov/media/9776/foodaps_datauserperspective.pdf.

Wilde, P., and Ranney, C.K. (2000). The monthly food stamp cycle: Shopping frequency and food intake decisions in an endogenous switching regression framework. *American Journal of Agricultural Economics, 82*(1), 200–213.

Wilde, P., Llobrera, J., and Ver Ploeg, M. (2014). Population density, poverty, and food retail access in the United States: An empirical approach. *International Food and Agribusiness Management Review, 17* (Special Issue A). https://www.ifama.org/resources/Documents/v17ia/Wilde-Llobrera-Ploeg.pdf.

Yen, S.T., Andrews, M., Chen, Z., Eastwood, D.B. (2008). Food Stamp Program participation and food insecurity: An instrumental variables approach. *American Journal of Agricultural Economics, 90*(1), 117–132.

Young, J. (2017). *The Differences in Characteristics among Households With and Without Obese Children: Findings from USDA's Food APS.* EIB-179. Available: http://www.ers.usda.gov/webdocs/publications/85028/eib-179.pdf.

Zablotsky, B., and Black, L.I. (2019). Concordance between survey-reported childhood asthma and linked Medicaid administrative records. *Journal of Asthma, 56*(3), 285–295. https://doi.org/10.1080/02770903.2018.1455854.

Zeballos, E., and Anekwe, T. (2018). *The Association Between Nutrition Information Use and the Healthfulness of Food Acquisitions.* ERS No. 247. Washington, DC: U.S. Department of Agriculture, Economic Research Service.

Zeballos, E., and Restrepro, B. (2018). *Adult Eating and Health Patterns: Evidence from the 2014–2016 Eating and Health Module of the American Time Use Survey.* Economic Information Bulletin No. 198. Available: https://www.ers.usda.gov/publications/pub-details/?pubid=90465.

Zeballos, E., Todd, J., and Restrepo, B. (2019). *Frequency and Time of Day that Americans Eat: A Comparison of Data from the American Time Use Survey and the National Health and Nutrition Examination Survey.* Available: https://www.ers.usda.gov/publications/pub-details/?pubid=93513.

Zhen, C., Taylor, J.L., Muth, M., and Leibtag, E. (2009). Understanding differences in self-reported expenditures between household scanner data and diary survey data: A comparison of Homescan and the Consumer Expenditure Survey. *Review of Agricultural Economics, 31*(3), 470–492. Available: https://academic.oup.com/aepp/article/31/3/470/8063.

Ziliak, J.P. (2016). *Modernizing SNAP Benefits.* Washington, DC: The Brookings Institution. Available: http://www.hamiltonproject.org/assets/files/ziliak_modernizing_snap_benefits.pdf.

Appendix A

Summary, First Meeting, April 16, 2018

A.1. OVERVIEW OF ERS'S VISION AND STRATEGY FOR IMPROVING DATA FOR FOOD AND NUTRITION POLICY RESEARCH

The panel's first open meeting,[1] held April 16, 2018, consisted of a set of overview presentations by the U.S. Department of Agriculture's (USDA's) Economic Research Service (ERS) staff describing current projects in the agency's Consumer Food Data System (CFDS) portfolio and outlining priorities going forward. Panel members and meeting participants were informed about key program initiatives, including: plans for a possible second iteration of ERS's National Household Food Acquisition and Purchase Survey (FoodAPS); plans to make greater use of proprietary data sources; and continued development of linkages across multiple data sources (survey and nonsurvey) and of supplemental modules to surveys conducted by other federal statistical agencies. Research highlights emerging from CFDS program initiatives were also summarized.

Following introductory comments by **Marianne Bitler**, the panel chair, meeting participants were welcomed by **Brian Harris-Kojetin**, director of the Committee on National Statistics, and **Monica Feit**, deputy director of the Division of Behavioral and Social Sciences and Education, who also described the National Academies' study process. During this opening session, ERS leadership provided an overview of the agency's vision and strategy for improving data for food and nutrition policy research and specified their goals and objectives for commissioning the study. **Mary Bohman**, admin-

[1]The meeting agenda appears at the end of this appendix.

istrator of ERS, outlined the blueprint for the current CFDS program—describing its components, organization, and purpose—and its operational context within the agency's mission: to inform and enhance public and private decision making on economic and policy issues related to agriculture, food, the environment, and rural development.[2] Within this ERS mission, the role of the Food Economics Division is to

- take stock of contemporary and anticipated food policy and program objectives and market trends and dynamics;
- develop the necessary data and information infrastructure to examine the evolving questions; and
- produce the right products and information for the Administration, the Congress, and the public on consumer food choice behaviors and outcomes such as nutrition and health.

Bohman stated that the mandate for the Food Economics Division is to build a comprehensive, integrated data system focusing on consumer data to efficiently deliver credible evidence for informing policy and to facilitate production of research findings so that they are in place when food and nutrition-related policy and program needs arise.

Bohman further raised the question, central to the panel's charge, of whether new kinds of data sources perform as needed, and to what extent they might replace, supplement, or complement current data sources, primarily surveys. She stated that the main task for the panel was to help the agency chart its course going forward, particularly how it can most effectively put to use its $80 million investments in research, statistics, and data. She argued that the panel's report would have a substantial influence on the agency's ERS research and data strategies.

Jay Variyam, division director, ERS, described the motivation, vision, and action guiding CFDS activity. The motivation: policy needs drive data investments. The vision: to build a comprehensive, integrated data system to efficiently deliver credible evidence for informing policy. And the action: to develop a multipronged data approach to meet research and policy needs.

The most important policy areas and questions facing the Food Economics Division identified by Variyam are these:

- *Diets, Nutrition, and Obesity*—What foods do households buy, how much do they pay, where do they shop, and what is the nutritional quality of these purchases?
- *Food and Nutrition Safety Net*—How are USDA's Supplemental Nutrition Assistance Program (SNAP) participants and low-income

[2] See https://www.ers.usda.gov/about-ers.

households similar or different when taking diet, nutrition, and obesity into account?

- *Changing Consumer Preferences*—How do consumers respond to price changes, new information, and varying product attributes?
- *Food Environment and Affordability*—What role does the food environment play in consumers' food choices? Does ease of access matter for the nutritional quality of purchases?
- *Industry Response and Changing Food Supply*—How is the food supply changing in response to consumer preferences for convenience, nutrition, and production attributes, and what are the nutritional implications?
- *Agricultural Sector Adaptations*—How will the agricultural sector adapt to changing consumer preferences, and what are the resource implications?

Echoing Bohman's comments, Variyam envisioned a multiple-data approach for the agency. Both beyond and in coordination with FoodAPS and other surveys, other forms of data will be involved, including proprietary scanner data, linked administrative data, food store data, and linked nutrition and food acquisition data. The motivation behind this multipronged data approach is that, even given the impressive amount (and quality) of data on food and food program participation that exists across federal statistical agencies, these sources are still insufficient to answer key questions about consumer choices, food acquisitions, industry response, and the role and effectiveness of government programs.

Mark Denbaly, deputy division director for Food Economics Data, ERS, elaborated on the multiple-data-source approach. In an era of increasing costs and decreasing public willingness to spend time completing surveys, proprietary and other alternative data are gaining in importance across the statistical system. Examples of this trend within the CFDS at ERS include use of the following:

- IRI household item-level data on grocery purchases,[3]
- IRI retail store item-level sales data,
- IRI product descriptions and attributes for about 1 million UPCs,
- Nielsen store characteristics and geocoded locations (TDLinx[4]), and
- NPD restaurant locations and characteristics (ReCount[5]).

[3] For more information on IRI products used by ERS, see https://www.ers.usda.gov/webdocs/publications/47633/57105_tb-1942.pdf?v=0.

[4] For more information, see https://www.nielsen.com/us/en/press-releases/2017/nielsen-tdlinx-announces-new-channel-classification-for-dining-industry.

[5] For more information, see https://www.npd.com/wps/portal/npd/us/news/press-releases/2018/total-us-restaurant-count-at-647288-a-drop-from-last-year-due-to-decline-in-independent-restaurant-units-reports-npd.

Integration across data sources is another key element of ERS's state data strategy. Among data-combining initiatives undertaken by the agency to date are these:

- integrating USDA's Agricultural Research Service (ARS) nutrient information with IRI scanner data, an interagency effort that also involves USDA's Center for Nutrition Policy (CNPP);
- using a geospatial data system to provide precise information about food retail environments; and
- linking agency administrative records to survey data—the purpose of the Next Generation Data Platform (as described in Chapter 2, this is an interagency effort with the Census Bureau and USDA's Food and Nutrition Services [FNS]).

A third element of ERS's CFDS strategy involves developing supplements to existing surveys. The agency has already had success with this strategy—for example, the Flexible Consumer Behavior Survey, which was added to the Centers for Disease Control and Prevention's (CDC's) National Health and Nutrition Examination Survey (NHANES),[6] the Eating and Health Module added to the Bureau of Labor Statistics' (BLS's) Time Use Survey, and the Food Security Module, which was added to CDC's National Health Interview Survey, and is open to greater use of modules where subject matter synergies arise.

Although covered in greater detail by other presenters, Denbaly provided a brief overview of FoodAPS. Designed in consultation with academic and government leaders and experts (and jointly sponsored with FNS), the survey

- integrates multiple types of information from multiple sources;
- brings together food, economics, nutrition, health, program participation, and environmental factors;
- focuses on food acquisition, not on food intake;
- is more than an expenditure study, as it includes prices and quantities of acquired food at the item level;
- includes acquisition of food items consumed at home and food items consumed away from home, as well as free foods; and
- is the only source of information on food items that participants acquire using program benefits and their own resources.[7]

[6] For more information, see https://www.ers.usda.gov/topics/food-choices-health/food-consumption-demand/flexible-consumer-behavior-survey.

[7] Additional details can be found at https://www.ers.usda.gov/foodaps.

A.2. DISCUSSION OF THE PROJECT STATEMENT OF TASK AND PRIORITIZATION OF TOPICS FOR THE STUDY

Following review by ERS leadership presentations, there was open discussion of the project Statement of Task and prioritization of topics for the study. Panel members provided their perspectives, identifying key issues embodied in the charge and discussing their primary interests related to the study. This discussion yielded the revised Statement of Task (see Chapter 1).

During discussion of the Statement of Task, Mark Denbaly noted the importance of identifying the most important policy questions to be answered; these questions, in turn, would drive how the division invested in its data infrastructure. Many of the thoughts on these issues are encapsulated in the above-referenced white paper produced by ERS for the panel. Denbaly asked that the panel consider the return on investment for various data infrastructure options. Panel members noted that "assessing the value" of different data investments requires identifying a cost/benefit metric—which might consider research-enabled use of data in program administration, amount of staff time, and dollar costs. These metrics are not readily available. All agreed that informing policy was a top priority.

A major question raised by Denbaly was what to do with FoodAPS. How can it be improved in regard to reduced burden and improved location and price information? Should future iterations of the survey be pursued and, if so, how should they be specified? And, what are the alternative uses of FoodAPS resources, and could these alternatives provide the same value to researchers and policy makers? To begin framing these questions, the next session consisted of presentations by ERS staff to inform panel members about current CFDS data programs, research activities, and program plans. The session was meant to stimulate panel thinking about what additional kinds of information the panel might need in order to carry out its charge.

A.3. CURRENT CFDS PROGRAMS, RESEARCH ACTIVITIES, AND PLANS

Kicking off a session on "Current data programs, research activities, and program plans," **David Levin** and **Megan Sweitzer**, both ERS economists, described use of proprietary data by the Food Economics Division. One prominent example is the use by the agency of data collected and processed by the company, IRI (https://www.iriworldwide.com/en-US/Company/About-Us). IRI collects proprietary scanner data on consumer purchase transactions, retail point-of-sales (purchase transaction records are collected from store systems), household scanner data for store purchases (which can be sometimes be linked with household demographics), and product and store information.[8]

Among the advantages of scanner data cited by Levin and Sweitzer is their granularity. Food price data can be pinpointed geographically to individual stores or market areas. Product detail is available at the level of each individual UPC/item, to which descriptions and attributes are attached. Data are often available on a weekly basis. Sample sizes are large, and in some cases long-term panels of households have been constructed.

Scanner data have been integrated more broadly across USDA into cost estimates and evaluations of USDA programs. Projects to estimate the weights of Special Supplemental Nutrition Program for Women, Infants, and Children (WIC) food packages and the retail value of the average Food Distribution Program on Indian Reservations (FDPIR) food package are two examples.

Limitations of scanner data noted by Levin and Sweitzer have to do with their representativeness and accessibility in a documented format. Future work could usefully be conducted on improving the representativeness of the retail data and developing weights for the retail stores. Creating a capacity to link stores in household and retail data would also be valuable, as would creating new identifiers/variables for SNAP and WIC purchases.

Indeed, ERS has plans in place to expand scanner data applications. One example is the Quarterly Food-at-Home Price Database (QFAHPD), which aggregates food purchases from Nielsen Homescan for more than 50 food groups (available to the public on the ERS website). Another is in future iterations of FoodAPS to support product identification and food environment studies. The panel was asked to weigh in on these issues in its report, to provide a sense of the way these different commercial datasets may be used in stand-alone applications by researchers, and in what ways they may be combined with survey or other nonsurvey data in the CFDS.

Andrea Carlson, ERS, elaborated on the project to integrate USDA's ARS nutrient information with IRI scanner data, an interagency effort also involving USDA's Center for Nutrition Policy and Promotion (CNPP) and ARS. The challenge is to create prices for foods consumed as collected by NHANES, preferably using automated methods, and to match them with nutrient data. The first step was to create a crosswalk, the Purchase-to-Plate Crosswalk, between purchased foods from scanner data (45,000 codes) and foods found in FNDDS (about 5,000 codes) and develop prices for foods reported on NHANES as consumed (8,000 items). The terms used for foods are different in the two sources. A semi-automatic approach has been tested with data from two time periods.

---

[8] A full description of ERS use of scanner and other kinds of commercial data can be found in Chapter 2.

The project also developed Food Purchase and Acquisition Food Groups (F-PAG)—now called ERS Food Purchase Groups (EFPG)—which assign IRI UPCs to USDA-related food groups, based on ingredients, nutritional content, and convenience to consumer and store aisle. An earlier version of this database is linked to Food-APS for studying the nutritional content of purchased foods and the F-PAG are similar to the groups used to prepare the Quarterly Food at Home Price Database. The project also created the Food and Nutrition Database for Dietary Study (FNDDS)[9] and the Purchase to Plate Price Tool, which estimates prices for individual foods consumed as reported in What We Eat in America (WWEIA) and NHANES. This tool supports analysis of the relationship between food prices and nutritional content.

The tools have been used to augment publicly available data from existing surveys. External users have restricted access to them. New external data products that resulted include these:

- *ERS Quarterly Food at Home Price Database (QFAHPD):* https://www.ers.usda.gov/data-products/quarterly-food-at-home-price-database/ERS
- *ERS Fruit and Vegetable Prices (FVP) data product:* https://www.ers.usda.gov/data-products/fruit-and-vegetable-prices.aspx
- *Food Consumption and Nutrient Intakes 2007–2010,* based on NHANES data: https://www.ers.usda.gov/data-products/food-consumption-and-nutrient-intakes/
- *Commodity Consumption by Population Characteristics 1994–2008,* using FADS and NHANES: https://www.ers.usda.gov/data-products/commodity-consumption-by-population-characteristics/

Next, **Michele (Shelly) Ver Ploeg**, chief of the Food Assistance Branch, ERS, presented options for linking survey data to food environment data. The motivation for these kinds of data linkages is to be able to address research questions concerning whether Americans' diets are out of balance with dietary guidelines and, if so, to what extent it is due to a lack of access to healthy and affordable foods and to what extent to the larger food environment (e.g., availability of stores and restaurants, variation in food prices, food policies, and community characteristics) that may influence food choices and diet quality.

To pursue the measurement of these accessibility issues, ERS has invested in proprietary food retailer and restaurant data, which have been combined

[9]FNDDS is a database maintained by Agricultural Research Service (ARS) that contains information on foods, their nutrient content values, and the weights of portions. It is used to analyze the nutrient content of foods consumed as reported in WWEIA/NHANES.

with survey and administrative data (e.g., population and food assistance program data) to produce food access and food environment indicators. Ver Ploeg described a number of products that have emerged from this initiative. One of these, the *Food Access Research Atlas*, provides a spatial overview of access to supermarkets, supercenters, and large grocery stores. Another, the *Food Environment Atlas*, distills more than 200 indicators of a community's ability to access healthy food and its success in doing so. The *Food Environment Atlas* includes county-level detail for most indicators, as well as indicators of store and restaurant availability, food assistance use, food prices and taxes, local foods initiatives, and health and physical activity.

ERS's data and mapping tools are used in research, in policy, and by planners. The FoodAPS geography component adapts the *Atlas* information in the construction of its survey instruments and to characterize the food retail environment in a given primary or secondary sampling unit. These data and mapping tools have also been linked to other surveys, including the IRI Consumer Panel, Panel Study of Income Dynamics (PSID), the Health and Retirement Study (HRS), NHANES, and CPS. Policy applications include the Healthy Food Finance Initiative (Treasury, HHS, USDA) and SNAP store authorization regulations. And, among community planners and local governments, the *Atlases* have consistently been among the ERS products with the greatest number of web views.

Mark Prell, ERS, presented information about the Next Generation Data Platform, which is a strategic partnership among ERS, Food and Nutrition Services, and the U.S. Census Bureau (Census) to promote record linking for research purposes. The platform is a long-term effort to acquire state-level administrative microdata for SNAP and WIC that can then be linked to Census survey data and administrative files from other federal agencies in a secure data environment to support research on USDA programs.

As articulated by Prell, the Next Generation Data Platform project goals are to inform policy makers, managers, and the public on (i) who participates in USDA food assistance programs; (ii) how participation affects people's lives; and (iii) who does not participate and why. The Census Bureau brings to the project the data infrastructure expertise to inform decisions regarding the use of surveys (including the 2020 Census), data-linkage processes and regulation, and linkage agreements with other federal agencies.

Among the benefits of SNAP administrative data are that they include information on the *universe* of SNAP participants in a given state and that these data are known for their completeness and accuracy. Among the benefits of American Community Survey (ACS) data are that they are a random sample of both SNAP and non-SNAP participants and include demographic information as well as annual income data—used to model SNAP income eligibility. The benefit of linking SNAP and ACS data is that the strength of each data source can be leveraged.

During the day's final open session, **Elina Page** of ERS presented on information about FoodAPS and plans for future iterations of the survey. She began by outlining the needs for a data source such as FoodAPS. The primary objective of the program is to inform policy on diet-related health issues, an important policy issue. The economic burden of diet-related diseases reaches into the trillions of dollars each year for the nation. For 2016, the cost of obesity and overweight conditions alone—in terms of direct expenditures and lost productivity—was estimated to be $1.42 trillion (Milken Institute, 2016; Benjamin et al., 2017). Cardiovascular diseases ($316 billion) and type 2 diabetes ($320 billion) are the two costliest condition categories.

Page pointed out that the high level of program spending to improve the population's health provides another pressing policy impetus for collecting accurate and timely information. In 2016, Medicare and Medicaid spending reached $672 billion and $566 billion, respectively. For 2017, expenditures on other key programs were as follows:

- all food assistance programs, $99 billion;
- SNAP, $68 billion (for an average monthly participation of 42 million);
- WIC, $6 billion (for an average monthly participation of 7 million);
- National School Lunch Program, $14 billion (for an average daily participation of 30 million); and
- National School Breakfast Program, $4 billion (for an average daily participation of 15 million (Oliveira, 2018).

Table A.1, from Page's presentation, lists key data sources for documenting these expenditures and their effectiveness at fulfilling their stated goals.

As indicated by gaps in Table A.1, it is clear that current information needs are met only incompletely. FoodAPS was designed to address these shortcomings by collecting comprehensive data on household food purchases and acquisitions; foods from food-at-home (FAH) retailers; food-away-from-home (FAFH) establishments; and foods obtained for free. Information is reported by all household members over a 7-day period during the period in which the survey was fielded (from April 2012 to January 2013).

Page described the FoodAPS sample as nationally representative of U.S. households with four target populations: (i) SNAP households, (ii) non-SNAP households with income < 100 percent of the federal poverty guideline, (iii) non-SNAP households with income ≥ 100 percent and < 185 percent of the federal poverty guideline, and (iv) non-SNAP households with income ≥ 185 percent of the federal poverty guideline. Table A.2 describes the composition of the FoodAPS participants in more detail.

Goals for future iterations of *FoodAPS* would be to capture higher quality data, reduce nonresponse bias, reduce respondent burden and reporting fatigue, and reduce processing time. A key strategy for accomplishing these

TABLE A.1 Data Sources

	SIPP (Survey of Income and Program Participation)	NHANES (National Health and Nutrition Examination Survey)	CE (Consumer Expenditure Survey)	Proprietary Consumer Panels
	Census	NCHS CDC	BLS	Nielsen Homescan or the IRI Consumer Network
Food-at-home purchases			⚠	✓
Food-away-from-home purchases			⚠	
Free food acquisitions				
Household unit	✓			✓
Food assistance program participation	✓	⚠	⚠	⚠
Demographics	✓	✓	✓	✓

✓ = included
⚠ = included with limitations
SOURCE: Presentation to the panel by Elina T. Page, April 16, 2018. Reprinted with permission.

TABLE A.2 Categories of FoodAPS Survey Participants

	Full Survey	SNAP Households	Non-SNAP + <100%	Non-SNAP + ≥100% + <185%	Non-SNAP + ≥185%
Households	4,826	1,581	346	851	2,048
Individuals	14,317	5,414	964	2,375	5,564
FAH Events	15.998	5,545	1,134	2,711	6,608
FAH Items	143,050	51,145	8,693	21,878	61,334
FAFH Events	39,120	12,371	2,311	6,329	18,109
FAFH Events	116,074	37,140	6,831	18,480	53,623

NOTES: SNAP = Supplemental Nutrition Assistance Program, FAH = food at home, FAFH = food away from home. "Events" are usually self-reported purchases and do not involve scanner data, while "items" are scanned purchases.
SOURCE: Presentation to the panel by Elina T. Page, April 16, 2018. Reprinted with permission.

goals is to continue exploring data linkage options. *FoodAPS* survey data are already linked to the extant data to reduce respondent burden and enhance data analysis. As described above, proprietary scanner data were used to create item descriptions and weights. SNAP administrative records were used in sampling frame and data quality checks. Thirteen data sources were used to enhance the *FoodAPS* geography component—specifically, to fill in details (location and density of retailers, measures of access to these retailers, local food prices, and area demographics) about the local food environments. Finally, the USDA food nutrient databases were used to add micro- and macro-nutrient content and food pattern equivalents to the *FoodAPS*-generated micro record.

Page concluded her presentation by posing the following questions for the panel to consider as it deliberates on its charge and, hopefully, to answer: Where is FoodAPS headed? Is FoodAPS worth the investment? And should FoodAPS be a permanent data collection effort?

A.4. MEETING AGENDA

Panel on Improving USDA's Consumer Data for Food and Nutrition Policy Research

The National Academy of Sciences Building, Lecture Room
2101 Constitution Ave. NW, Washington, DC

Meeting Goals: The panel's first meeting consists of a set of high-level overview presentations by ERS staff about current projects and priorities of the agency's Consumer Food Data System (CFDS) program. These presentations will inform panel members, and meeting participants more broadly, about key developments—exploiting proprietary data, developing linkages across disparate data sources, adding supplements to exiting surveys, and continued planning for FoodAPS-2—pushing forward the CFDS data infrastructure. Research highlights emerging from various CFDS program initiatives will also be summarized. During this afternoon closed session, the panel will review (and, if necessary, refine) its charge, attend to institutional requirements, and finalize planning of an open session for the project's second meeting in June.

Open Public Sessions, 9:00 a.m.–3:00 p.m.

9:00 Welcome, introductions, and overview of agenda
- **Marianne Bitler**, *Chair*
- **Brian Harris-Kojetin**, *Director, Committee on National Statistics*
- **Monica Feit**, *Deputy Director, DBASSE*

9:30 Sponsor's welcome; high-level overview of the agency's vision and strategy for improving data for food and nutrition policy research
Goals and objectives of the study (20 minutes)
- **Mary Bohman,** *Administrator, ERS*; **Jay Variyam,** *Division Director, ERS*

Blueprint for the current CFDS program—components, organization, and rationale
- **Mark Denbaly,** *Deputy Division Director for Food Economics Data, ERS*

Questions from the panel; general discussion (20 minutes)

10:45 Discussion of the project *Statement of Task* and prioritization of topics for the study
- **Panel members'** perspectives: each panel member identifies key issues embodied in the charge and discusses primary interests related to the study (5 minutes each)
- Response from **sponsors** and open discussion (15 minutes)

1:00 Current data programs, research activities, and program plans. More detailed presentations by ERS staff to inform panel members about CFDS program activities. The session should also be oriented to stimulate panel thinking about what kinds of presentations would be most useful to pursue during the open portion of meeting #2.

Session 1: Use of proprietary data (25 minutes, 15 minutes Q&A)
- **David Levin** and **Megan Sweitzer,** *Economists, ERS*

Session 2: Other non-survey data sources
Linking to nutrition information (10 minutes)
- **Andrea Carlson,** *Economist, ERS*

Linking to food environment data (10 minutes)
- **Shelly Ver Ploeg** *Chief, Food Assistance Branch, ERS*

Next Generation Data Platform for Administrative Data (10 minutes)
- **Mark Prell,** *Senior Economist, ERS*

Questions from the panel; general discussion (10 minutes)

Session 3: FoodAPS-1 and Plans for FoodAPS-2 (25 minutes, 15 minutes Q&A)
- **Elina Page,** *Economist, ERS*

3:00 p.m. *Adjourn*

Appendix B

Summary, Second Meeting, June 14, 2018

The panel's second meeting included presentations covering a range of topics integral to addressing the study charge, including the current and potential use of proprietary commercial and other nongovernmental, nonsurvey data sources; users' perspectives on directions for Economic Research Service's (ERS's) National Household Food Acquisition and Purchase Survey (FoodAPS) survey; and the linking of data sources. The topics covered in the four sessions, which align with this summary, were: (i) proprietary data used by (or of interest to) ERS; (ii) combining data sources to advance food and nutrition policy and research; (iii) use of specialized modules added to federal surveys; and (iv) a FoodAPS-2 status update along with the perspectives of data users and stakeholders.

B.1. PROPRIETARY DATA USED BY (OR OF INTEREST TO) ERS

After introductory comments by the panel chair, **Marianne Bitler**, and by **Jay Variyam** and **Mark Denbaly** of ERS, the panel heard from presenters about proprietary data. This session built on the April 16, 2018, presentation by **Megan Sweitzer** and **David Levin** (both of ERS) on the same topic. Proprietary data from commercial data sources may supplement (and, in some cases, replace) survey data. Sources of proprietary (purchased) data used by ERS include these:

- *TDLinx, Nielsen* (2004–2017)—Names and geospatial locations of food stores in the United States with sales greater than $1 million; used in ERS geospatial database;

- *ReCount, NPD Group* (1998–2017)—Locations and characteristics of restaurants; used in ERS geospatial database;
- *IRI Consumer Network* (2008–2017)—Household panel data, including scanner data (also includes MedProfiler and RXPulse, two household health surveys), and Nielsen Homescan (1998–2010)—Household panel data, including scanner data used in the ERS Quarterly Food at Home Price Database;
- *IRI InfoScan* (2007–2017)—Retail scanner data; used in the ERS Quarterly Food at Home Price Database; and
- *Nielsen Homescan* (1998–2010)—Household panel data, including scanner data.

Kicking off the meeting, **Abigail Okrent** (ERS) described ERS's work to use proprietary commercial data and to understand its strengths and weaknesses. Okrent reported that ERS purchases household panel data (including scanner data) because they offer several advantages. The Consumer Network Panel is used by both Nielsen and IRI in their commercial household panel products. The panel has a large sample size, more than 120,000 households, with around half of these households providing purchase data. Additionally, the same households can participate in the panel every year. Researchers are able to append geographic food environment and economic information from other datasets to household-level records so the impacts of the food environment or macroeconomic conditions on household purchasing patterns can be examined. Scanner information is collected at the UPC level, which conveys brand, type, and manufacturer information; and household geographic location can be identified down to the census tract level.

To evaluate the strengths and limitations of proprietary household panel data, ERS has collaborated with colleagues from RTI[1] and academic institutions on a number of studies. In reviewing these studies, Okrent pointed out two common concerns. The first is that households are not randomly selected into the panel and, hence, the sample might not be representative of the population. Second, households that agree to participate in the sample might not record all of their purchases or might not record them correctly.

Okrent summarized some validation studies. Einav, Leibtag, and Nevo (2008) matched Nielsen Homescan households' purchase records with data obtained from a large grocery retailer. The authors found that 80 percent of food-shopping trips in Nielsen Homescan showed up in the store's data; the unmatched trips likely resulted from households not reporting all of their trips. For matched trips they found that about 93 percent of the time the two data sources reported the same quantity. The reported expenditure was the same about 49 percent of the time.

---

[1] See https://www.rti.org.

A study by Sweitzer and colleagues (2017) compared weighted expenditures in the IRI Consumer Panel with the Consumer Expenditure Survey (CES) and FoodAPS by food subcategories and demographic groups. The results from this study show that expenditures in the IRI data were lower than expenditures in the CES, but the magnitude and variation of these differences varied across food categories, years, and household demographic characteristics. Many of the food categories with the most underreporting are those that contain more random-weight products (e.g., fruits and vegetables that are measured by the pound).

These comparison studies suggest that researchers should be cautious when using the IRI household data for certain types of studies, such as research focusing on fresh fruits and vegetables or high-income or large households and studies that draw conclusions about the overall composition of consumers' purchases or diets.

The strength of commercial scanner data, both for households and retail, is the detail they can provide on nutrition facts labeling information (e.g., calories, sodium, and calcium per package); health and nutrition-related claims (e.g., whether gluten-free, type of sugar/artificial sweetener, whole grain claims); and other claimed characteristics (e.g., organic, no preservative, hormone-free, natural).

The strengths of store data, such as InfoScan, are realized from highly detailed information on weekly food purchases for large numbers of stores; expenditures and quantities of UPC and random-weight food products; and location of establishments. Similarly, store characteristics data sources, such as TDLinx, National Economic Time Series (NETS),[2] and ReCount, offer detail on retail and food service establishments, including location and sales and employment information for each store.

ERS research (Levin et al., 2018) has compared store counts across TDLinx, NETS, and InfoScan.[3] For the period of 2008–2012, the authors found that the number of stores and food sales in InfoScan were considerably lower than those in TDLinx and NETS. Comparing these totals to the 2012 Economic Census indicates that the version of InfoScan purchased by ERS covered about half of all sales.

Okrent reported that ERS is currently working on solutions to alleviate shortcomings in their application of commercial data. They are using available data to develop weights or projection factors to use to help make the store-level data more representative and for imputing missing random-weight prices.

---

[2]The National Economic Time Series database is available from Willis and Associates. It is based on establishment information from Dunn and Bradstreet.

[3]Okrent pointed out that InfoScan only releases data to ERS for stores that agree to this arrangement, and this is limited to stores that make more than $2 million in sales. Also, some stores only release their sales data for their retail marketing area, which is retailer-defined.

Brian Burke of IRI described the company's point-of-sale data, which InfoScan collects on a weekly basis from more than 200,000 stores globally. The company's IRI Consumer Network Panel includes more than 110,000 consumers. The company has some health and wellness data in these databases now and will be expanding that feature in the future. IRI also has a shopper loyalty database with more than 125 million loyalty card holders. Finally, the company offers analytics that leverage its data assets.

Ann Hanson and **Louis Lesce** of the NPD Group summarized their data products, noting that they have point-of-sale data from retailers, distributors, and food service operators and that they also conduct consumer surveys. NPD Group has a number of food industry databases, and Hanson and Lesce summarized four: National Eating Trends, NPD's consumer database with 19,000 respondents and food consumption data for at-home and away-from-home eating; Eating Patterns in America, NPD's annual analysis of the state of food and drink consumption in the United States with long-term and emerging trends; ReCount (used by ERS), a census of food service locations (650,000 restaurants, 130,000 convenience stores, and 450,000 noncommercial locations); and CREST, another consumer database, which has 440,000 buyers and focuses on consumer use of food service establishments for meals, snacks, or drinks. With its food databases, NPD Group provides research on food consumption, restaurants, and commercial food service and eating patterns. The firm is working on adding nutrient intake to National Eating Trends and are working on analysis of local market data using CREST.

Joseph Fortson of Nielsen observed that shopper consumer behavior has changed over the years, and data such as Homescan and TDLinx (both used or formerly used by ERS) can be used to quantify those changes and help firms take advantage of trends. He noted the rise in online shopping and commented that one issue online vendors face is the alignment and coherence (or lack thereof) between federal and state regulations.

During open discussion, panel member **Craig Gunderson** pointed out the tendency of sources such as Homescan to underrepresent low-income consumers. He suggested that it would be useful to researchers if the number of low-income households could be increased in the Homescan data, especially in some of their longitudinal panels. Fortson pointed out that Nielsen does aggressively recruit in lower-income and diverse areas, because they are the toughest populations to capture. Burke noted that IRI surveys tend to rely on participants "opting in" but that they do target difficult-to-reach groups and the data are weighted to be representative of the population. Lesce stated that NPD has considered redirecting some surveys to specific demographics. For example, they already have a Hispanic consumer survey. Fortson noted that incentives to participate in proprietary surveys in the form of payments (albeit small ones) mean more to low-income families than they do to high-income families.

B.2. COMBINING DATA SOURCES TO ADVANCE FOOD AND NUTRITION POLICY AND RESEARCH

One example of a combined data source is the USDA Branded Food Products Database, described by **Alison Krester** of ILSI International, a nonprofit science foundation that is primarily funded by the food and beverage industry, and **Kyle McKillop** of the University of Maryland. This data source augments the USDA National Nutrient Database[4] with nutrient composition and ingredient information on branded and store-brand food products provided by the food industry. The Branded Food Products Database project is a public-private partnership initiated by former undersecretary of USDA, Catherine Woteki. The goal of the project is to enhance public health and the sharing of open data.

The USDA Branded Food Products Database (BFPDB)—since 2019, the USDA Global Branded Food Products Database—covers 229,064 branded products from 238 food categories. Data elements include product name and generic descriptor; serving size in grams or milliliters; nutrients on the Nutrition Facts Panel per serving size and on a 100-gram basis, 100 milliliter basis, or fluid-ounce basis; ingredient list (never before captured by USDA); and date stamp associated with most current product formulation.

Linking the BFPDB to specific years of National Health and Nutrition Examination Survey (NHANES) surveys, if possible, could more accurately assess dietary intake within the United States. Having a historical record of branded and private-label foods enables comparisons of current and past consumption. Having a historical record of branded and private-label foods enables comparisons of current and past consumption. The BFPDB is in the public domain and is accessible through an Application Programing Interface (API) or directly through the Internet, where users can search, filter, and export their results.

Krester and McKillop argued that this initiative marks a paradigm shift for USDA—and that the benefit to the research community of gaining a large amount of data from food manufacturers on their food products may be a more efficient and cost-effective way of obtaining data than the usual survey approach. Next steps for the project include continuing to grow the database and creating awareness to increase its use. There are also plans for global expansion, as well as to add restaurant foods and food service products, increase private-label food items, and add foods imported into the United States. Work will also continue to align a standardized, validated algorithm to be used across all food products to determine food groupings.

---

[4]The USDA National Nutrient Database and the USDA Branded Foods Database are part of USDA's Food Composition Databases. See https://ndb.nal.usda.gov/ndb.

Next, building on the theme of combining data sources, **Biing-Hwan Lin** of ERS discussed a project linking ERS's Food Availability Data System (FADS)[5] to nutrition intake data from the Agricultural Research Service (ARS).[6] FADS measures food commodity supplies from the farmer to domestic consumption. The central motivation behind the project is to be able to develop value-added data products that can be used to analyze both intakes and density of foods and nutrients by food source and population characteristics, as well as to measure commodity consumption by food source and population characteristics.

The project described by Lin combined food consumption data from NHANES for 2007–2010 with USDA's Food Patterns Equivalents Database (FPED, formerly known as MyPyramid Equivalents Database) to estimate food consumption by food groups, as specified in the 2010 *Dietary Guidelines for Americans*. For example, a respondent in NHANES may report having eaten a specific amount of apple pie; this piece of data is then mapped into other measures such as cups of fruit, ounces of grain, grams of oils and solid fat, and teaspoons of added sugars (the commodities that make up apple pie). The consumption and nutrient content are reported by food source and can be summarized according to respondents' demographic characteristics. In a collaborative effort with ERS and the National Center for Health Statistics (NCHS), ARS has converted the NHANES and USDA consumption intake data into 65 agricultural commodities. This Food Intakes Converted to Retail Commodities Database (FICRCD) includes retail-level commodities that fall into eight categories: dairy products; fats and oils; fruits; grains; meat, poultry, fish, and eggs; nuts; caloric sweeteners; and vegetables, dry beans, and legumes. This information was leveraged to convert ERS's loss-adjusted food availability data (the "consumption" part of FADS), into the 65 agricultural commodities by age, income, ethnicity, and region for both food at home and food away from home.

Lin concluded by laying out data needs along with the future work plan for the project. One such data need is for farmers to better understand who consumes their commodity, where it is consumed, and how it is served. As noted above, the food consumption survey covers food (e.g., apple pie), but not at the commodity level (apples). For the loss-adjusted food availability database, future work includes building in more timely updates, expanding the number of commodities in the FICRCD, and converting food acquisition to retail commodities databases for FoodAPS (databases that capture purchases rather than consumption.)

[5] See https://www.ers.usda.gov/data-products/food-availability-per-capita-data-system.

[6] Andrea Carlson described another ERS project involving the ARS nutrient databases during the first workshop.

During open discussion, panel member **Jim Ziliak** asked what the mission directive was underlying the choice of the 65 agricultural commodities. Lin responded that category design was driven by the sample size. If there were a sufficient number of observations, the food was assumed to have been eaten quite frequently in the marketplace, and so it could be included in the commodity list. But if there were not enough observations—for example, to separate out almonds from tree nuts—then the food item remained in the more highly aggregated group.

B.3. USE OF SPECIALIZED MODULES ADDED TO FEDERAL SURVEYS

ERS has actively expanded its Consumer Food Data System (CFDS) by sponsoring or cosponsoring modules on surveys conducted by other agencies. These include the Food Security Supplement, added to many surveys, the Flexible Consumer Behavior Survey (FCBS), which has been added to NHANES, and the Eating and Health Module (EHM), added to the Bureau of Labor Statistics' American Time Use Survey (ATUS).

Eliana Zeballos of ERS provided an overview of the EHM call out supplement to the ATUS. She said that implementation of the EHM was motivated by the need for information about individuals' decisions on how to use their time, which can have short- and long-run implications for income and earnings, health, and other aspects of well-being. The EHM collects data to analyze relationships associated with time use, eating behavior, obesity, and other health outcomes for important subpopulations such as SNAP and WIC participants, grocery shoppers, and meal preparers. Module questions fall into the following categories: eating and drinking as a secondary activity, grocery shopping and food-away from home (FAFH) purchases, meal preparation, food sufficiency and food assistance, household income, and height, weight, and general health.

Understanding time-use patterns can provide insight into economic behaviors associated with eating patterns as well as the diet and health status of individuals. Understanding whether participants in food and nutrition assistance programs face time constraints that differ from those of nonparticipants can inform the design of food assistance and nutrition policies and programs.

The EHM has supported a number of studies along these lines. One example of findings from this literature: Zeballos and Restrepo (2018) (see also Zeballos, Todd, and Restrepo, 2019) estimate that 58.2 percent of Americans ages 18 and older reported purchasing FAFH at some point during the week before their interview. About 43 percent of individuals who received SNAP benefits in the past month made a FAFH purchase. Another finding is that about 48 percent of individuals who received SNAP benefits had consumed a soft drink, which is 16.6 percent higher than the share of low-income, non-SNAP individuals who had done so.

Brandon Restrepo of ERS provided an overview of the FCBS, which has been fielded since 2007. The survey is "flexible" in the sense that it changes according to federal agency needs for timely, policy-relevant data. The FCBS includes a number of economic measures, including monthly income, assets, food expenditures, and participation in food and nutrition assistance programs (SNAP and WIC). It also includes dietary and behavioral measures, including self-assessed diet quality; use of packaged food labels when grocery shopping; importance of price, nutrition, and taste when grocery shopping or eating out; frequency of eating out; use of nutrition information on restaurant menus when eating out; and awareness of MyPlate and knowledge of calorie intake needs to maintain current weight.

FCBS data are valuable for informing policy evaluations of federal regulations on food labeling and its use by and impact on consumers. Restrepo concluded by stating that the goal of the FCBS going forward is to continue as a key add-on to the NHANES capable of providing timely national data to inform food and nutrition policy-making decisions.

Alisha Coleman-Jensen of ERS provided an overview of the Food Security Survey Module, describing different versions that have been used and the federal surveys onto which it has been added.[7] She also discussed research applications of the module.

Coleman-Jensen said that a typical definition of food insecurity stipulates that the household is unable, at some time during the year, to provide adequate food for one or more of its members due to a lack of resources. In an attempt to measure this, food security survey modules have employed various structures that vary in terms of the number of items/questions (e.g., 6, 10, or 18 items), whether child items are included or not, and by reference period (e.g., 12 months or 30 days). The main federal surveys in the U.S. Household Food Security Monitoring and Research System are the Current Population Survey Food Security Supplement (CPS); the American Housing Survey (AHS); the Early Childhood Longitudinal Surveys (ECLS); FoodAPS; NHANES; the National Health Interview Survey (NHIS); the Panel Study of Income Dynamics (PSID); the Survey of Income and Program Participation (SIPP); the Survey of Program Dynamics (SPD) and a growing number of state, local, and regional studies.[8]

Going forward, Coleman-Jensen stated that ERS continues to do research on the measure. For example, ERS is assessing the Spanish-language translation and assessing comparability for households with and without children. It is also conducting Rasch analyses to assess the measurement properties of the module in all federal surveys.

---

[7] See https://www.ers.usda.gov/topics/food-nutrition-assistance/food-security-in-the-us.

[8] For more information on these surveys in the context of ERS's CFNDS, see http://ers.usda.gov/data-products/food-security-in-the-united-states/documentation.aspx.

TABLE B.1 Planned Sample Size and Proposed Caseload for the Full Survey

Analytic Domain	Effective Sample Size	Proposed Number of Completed Cases
SNAP households	912	1,452
WIC households	606	739
Households with income-to-poverty ratios at or below 130% that do not participate in SNAP or WIC	895	1,426
Households with income-to-poverty ratios at or above 130% that do not participate in SNAP or WIC	876	1,824
All households	941	5,000

SOURCE: Data from ERS. Reprinted with permission.

B.4. FOODAPS-2 STATUS; DATA USERS' AND STAKEHOLDERS' INPUT

The afternoon session kicked off with an update from **Laurie May** and **Tom Krenzke** of Westat, the company contracted to design and field FoodAPS-2. The overarching objective in the planning for this second generation FoodAPS vehicle is to support new analyses, including broader analyses of USDA programs, and to improve data quality. This involves changes in the survey's sampling plan, instruments, and data collection procedures.

May and Krenzke identified the planned sample size for the full survey, as indicated in Table B.1.

These target figures are roughly comparable to those achieved for FoodAPS-1, which collected data from a sample of 4,826 households and is nationally representative. The survey targeted four groups, defined in terms of participation in SNAP and total reported household income.[9] Sampling plan changes from FoodAPS-1 involved increasing the WIC domain's effective sample size and creating WIC/SNAP likely-eligible flags. Other goals included improving data on children (by increasing representation) and implementing year-round data collection.

Planned changes to the survey instrument included the addition of questions covering

- more accurate school meal program information, including degree of daily participation and participation in summer meals program;
- food security (through an 18-question battery);
- subjective food needs;

[9] For exact figures, see https://www.ers.usda.gov/data-products/foodaps-national-household-food-acquisition-and-purchase-survey/documentation.

- food sensitivities and health conditions such as diabetes, high blood pressure, and high cholesterol;
- work schedule;
- online food purchasing; and
- improved geographic data, including travel distances to stores and restaurants and geocodes for residences and food places.

May and Krenzke also described planned data collection changes. To improve the overall completeness of data collection, Westat has been working to streamline the food log data input process for respondents, add look-up databases for items, and use reminders, targeted calls, and receipts to reduce underreporting of food acquisitions. To reduce respondent burden, Westat planned to replace hard-copy food logs with electronic food logs and income worksheets. To help achieve sample size goals and reduce nonresponse bias, Westat is planning to capture interviewer observations, implement an adaptive survey design, and improve imputation for missing items.

Parke Wilde and **Mehreen Ismail** of Tufts University presented findings from their work collecting user feedback from researchers using FoodAPS-1.[10] Wilde and Ismail reviewed 25 publications that presented results from FoodAPS, then surveyed 24 research teams that used the data. The literature review and data user survey demonstrated how FoodAPS has filled data gaps about food access and nutritional quality of food choices. Both information sources revealed that researchers largely were motivated to use FoodAPS for its high-quality, detailed coverage of food acquisitions and purchases, the food retail environment, and SNAP participation. However, it also revealed some limitations in data coverage and data quality. The specific needs identified include improvements needed in documentation, data files, and data access.

Next, **Robert Moffitt** of Johns Hopkins University added his assessment of the value of FoodAPS, which he called "a tremendous dataset in terms of breadth and the domain of the different types of questions related to the population's food consumption, nutrition, and health and on programs affecting on them." Moffitt's work relevant to FoodAPS has mainly concerned the impact of the SNAP program on various kinds of outcomes. His comments were in part methodological—specifically on how to establish and measure causal effects of participation in SNAP. Currently, FoodAPS, as a cross-sectional data source, is fairly limited in this regard, in comparison to the monitoring functions that a longitudinal dataset can serve. Most of the literature attempting to establish the causal impact of

[10] See *Review of the National Household Food Acquisition and Purchase Survey (FoodAPS) from a Data User's Perspective* at https://www.ers.usda.gov/media/9776/foodaps_datauserperspective.pdf.

food stamp participation on outcomes either uses panel data (where people moving into and out of the program can be observed) or applies some form of difference-in-differences analysis comparing people in different states or where the context is changing (e.g., the SNAP rules, eligibility conditions, or benefit levels, or even just the context of the economic conditions that may be inducing people to go on and off SNAP). This kind of analysis is difficult, because there are many other differences across states at a single point in time other than the food stamp benefit or other topic of analysis.

One of Moffitt's recommendations was that the FCNDS work toward more effective reconciliation of the SNAP program administrative datasets and the FoodAPS survey datasets. That, he said, would help alleviate difficulties in analyzing reporting errors with FoodAPS-1. He suggested that FoodAPS-2 use the same states as FoodAPS-1, especially those states that have validation data. He also suggested that ERS try to acquire SNAP histories for panel analysis.

Moffitt went on to say that reporting errors have not necessarily affected the bottom line result of policy interest—the question of whether SNAP affects outcomes or not, and by how much. Moffitt's conclusion was that the findings about the impact of SNAP on diet quality, food expenditure, food insecurity, obesity, the Healthy Eating Index (HEI), and so on are not very different whether the input data are from FoodAPS, administrative data, or some combination of the two sources.

Panel member **Diane Schanzenbach** suggested that much could be accomplished by improving the CPS the Consumer Expenditure Survey, or NHANES. She asked whether there is anything that suggests how measures of SNAP (or other program participation) could be improved on these surveys. She asked Moffitt why having a separate FoodAPS is better than improving the other larger, long-standing surveys.

Moffitt replied that what FoodAPS has that the other surveys do not have are the outcome measures: the nutritional measures, the diet quality measures, the HEI, the obesity measures and food expenditures. He noted that NHANES has very small sample sizes, perhaps even smaller than FoodAPS.

Someone in the audience commented that NHANES has health and nutrition outcomes but no economic outcomes. The Consumer Expenditure Survey has economic outcomes but no nutrition information. FoodAPS is basically the only survey that can link food, nutrition, economics, and health.

Next, **Susan Krebs-Smith** of the National Cancer Institute spoke about the use of data from USDA's Consumer Food Data System for health research. Her main topic was the HEI, designed to assess diet quality by showing how well any set of foods comports with the *Dietary Guidelines for Americans*. Krebs-Smith noted that part of USDA's mission is to ensure the healthfulness of the U.S. food supply. USDA is a partner in developing the *Dietary Guidelines for Americans*.

The HEI consists of 13 food group components (total fruits, whole fruits, total vegetables, greens and beans, whole grains, dairy, total protein foods, seafood and plant proteins, fatty acids, refined grains, sodium, added sugars, and saturated fats). Weights for constructing the index are derived from the *Dietary Guidelines*. The index requires information on the quantities of all of the food groups to generate the total score. It captures the balance among food groups, including foods to encourage and foods to reduce.

In addition to a total score, there is a score on each of the components. If the total HEI score is 100, all of the components are at their optimal level. If the total score is zero, every component is zero or very low. If the total score is, say, 55 (a very common score), the significance is not clear—for example, it remains unknown whether the diet is high on meats and low on vegetables, or vice versa.

One advantage of the HEI is that scores can be constructed at different levels in the food supply chain, from the commodities produced by farmers to the foods consumed by ultimate consumers and anything in between. In order to examine the HEI at different levels of the food chain, the foods or commodities at that level need to be identified and classified into the 13 categories of the HEI. Earlier during the day's meeting, **Biing-Hwan Lin** described translating the data from the ERS food supply system, FADS. With his apple pie example, he explained the difference between foods as eaten (like apple pie), commodities (apples), and the nutrients associated with them. For some levels of the food chain, that linkage can be done by using databases maintained and updated by ARS in collaboration with others. Constructing the HEI for FADS requires data from both the Nutrient Availability Database and the U.S. Salt Institute. Constructing the HEI for food consumption data from NHANES requires the Food Patterns Equivalent Database and the Nutrient Database. Crosswalk databases are still needed for food processing establishments and for the community food environment.

With the appropriate crosswalks, the HEI can be used to evaluate the "diet quality" associated with grocery store purchases, grocery store circulars, where food is obtained (e.g., different kinds of restaurants or fast food outlets), schools, food pantries, and so on. Also, in addition to using the index for comparison and monitoring, it could be used to analyze the relationships between diet patterns and health outcomes.

Krebs-Smith noted that the HEI provides a standardized measure across multiple levels and thinks this has real advantages. Making food comparable and available at all levels will involve overcoming some infrastructure challenges, which she thinks would be most useful to do.

Melissa Abelev of the Food and Nutrition Service (FNS) noted that FNS administers the USDA hunger programs: SNAP, WIC, the Child and Adult Care Food Program (CACFP), and the School Lunch and School Breakfast programs. FNS analysis groups provide cost data for budget analyses, analyzing how policy changes might impact the cost of food in FNS programs, how they might affect participation in the program, and how they might impact the overall cost of the program. They look at food security, the alignment of diets with nutritional standards, and program integrity and operations. They use a range of ERS and other data sources, including those of the Census Bureau and Bureau of Labor Statistics.

FNS has helped to fund a number of ERS initiatives, including FoodAPS and adding the Food Security Module to a variety of surveys. Abelev noted that FNS has not used FoodAPS data, however, primarily because the data are not user-friendly. FNS hopes to be able to use these data in the future, or to be better able to use the data from FoodAPS-2.

Following up on many of these themes, during open discussion participants discussed the strengths and weaknesses of using FoodAPS, and ideas for making future iterations more powerful. Panel member **Eric Rimm** pointed out that by the time FoodAPS-2 comes out, the online purchasing environment will have changed and become even more complex. Online shopping will become an important form of food acquisition. **Laurie May** and **Tom Krenzke** agreed, noting that they think in 2 years most food items will be available online. They stated that the online questionnaires had not yet been finalized, but agreed that nuances needed to be taken into account. At the event level, they will likely ask whether the purchase was online, delivered, or picked up in a grocery store. They will also collect information on items purchased.

Panel member **Amy O'Hara** asked about plans for broader use of data matching, specifically matching FoodAPS-2 to administrative data such as SNAP, WIC, Medicare, and Social Security data. May replied that Westat plans to use WIC and SNAP as part of the sampling plan. They are not currently planning to bring in other datasets. **Mark Denbaly** of ERS noted that simply getting ahold of SNAP and WIC data and matching them requires a heroic effort. O'Hara noted that ERC could buy Medicaid data and should consider how linkages might be facilitated several years down the road.

B.5. MEETING AGENDA

Panel on Improving USDA's Consumer Data for Food and Nutrition Policy Research
Second Meeting, June 14, 2018

The National Academy of Sciences Building, Room 120
2101 Constitution Ave NW, Washington, DC

<u>Meeting Goals:</u> The panel's second meeting will include a number of presentations geared toward informing the panel as it considers its charge and begins shaping a strategy for producing a report that fully addresses it.

Topics of interest for this meeting are the current and potential use of commercial and other non-government, non-survey data sources; users' perspectives on directions for ERS's FoodAPS survey; and linking data sources. Meeting #3 will follow up further on some of these topics. During closed session, the panel will review its charge, begin shaping a report outline, and identify key topics to address during its Fall meeting.

Day 1, June 14: Open Public Sessions

8:30 *Registration and networking; light breakfast available.*

9:00 Welcome, introductions, overview of agenda, goals for the meeting and the study
- **Marianne Bitler**, *Chair*
- **Jay Variyam, Mark Denbaly**, ERS

9:15 **Proprietary data used by (or of interest to) ERS**
This session will build on the April 16 presentation by **Megan Sweitzer** and **David Levin** (ERS). Commercial data sources can supplement (and, in some cases, replace) survey data, and CFDS program planners would like to explore the potential for increasing the use of commercial, web-based, and other non-survey data. Goals of a multi-source approach include reducing costs and respondent burden, increasing granularity or timeliness of information, and filling data gaps. ERS uses, or has used, consumer data from IRI, NPD, and Nielsen. Questions for presenters from commercial data firms include: How are data collected? What are the coverage and characteristics of the data? How are their data currently being used for research and policy? What access limitations and privacy issues affect data use? And, What is the level of transparency of methods to outside users? Presenters should identify data products they produce or plan to produce that may be of interest to statistical agencies.

- **Overview of commercial data currently used by ERS/CFDS program; ideas for expanding its use.** ERS is doing some creative work to estimate food prices to construct food plans. How are the quality and properties of data they are bringing into their program being evaluated (analogous to OMB quality standards for surveys)? What are the strengths and weaknesses of the data currently being used?
  - **Abigail Okrent**, ERS

- **IRI.** IRI is a big data analytics firm that collects information applicable to food policy research. Of particular interest to ERS are proprietary household and retail scanner price data (e.g., InfoScan) and also data on nutrition information and health and wellness claims for a large number of products.
  - **Brian Burke,** IRI (15 minutes)
- **NPD Group.** NPD collects consumer spending and consumption data across 3 main datasets, comprising direct point-of-sales feeds from retailers, consumer survey data and a receipt-based service, across 24+ sectors. With its food databases, NPD provides research on food consumption, restaurants, commercial food service, and eating patterns.
  - **Ann Hanson, Louis Lesce,** NPD
- **Nielsen.** ERS has used Nielsen Homescan and TDLinx data. TDLinx is a store/outlet-level database of retailers selling consumer packaged goods, including food.
  - **Joseph Fortson,** Nielsen
- Panel questions and comments, open discussion

10:45 **Combining data sources to advance food and nutrition policy and research**

- The USDA Branded Food Products Database. This data source augments the USDA National Nutrient Database with nutrient composition and ingredient information on branded and store-brand food products provided by the food industry.
  - **Alison Krester,** ILSI North America (30 minutes)
  - **Kyle McKillop,** University of Maryland, JIFSAN
- Linking the Food Availability Data System (FADS) to nutrition intake data from the Agricultural Research Service and National Center for Health Statistics to monitor and research the health and dietary outcomes of the U.S. population.
  - **Biing-Hwan Lin,** ERS (20 minutes)
- Panel questions and comments, open discussion

11:45 **Use of specialized modules added to federal surveys**

- The Eating and Health Module (EHM) supplement to the BLS American Time Use Survey, the Flexible Consumer Behavior Survey (FCBS), and other plans/opportunities for using the modules.
  - **Brandon Restrepo, Eliana Zeballos,** ERS (15 minutes)

- The Food Security Survey Module—how many versions are used (number of items and reference period) and what federal surveys has it been added to? What are the research applications?
  - **Alisha Coleman-Jensen,** ERS (15 minutes)
  - Panel questions and comments (Jay Breidt, Bruce Meyer, Eric Rimm); open discussion

1:30 **FoodAPS status; Data users' and stakeholders' input.** After a progress report on FoodAPS-2, participants will discuss the strengths and weaknesses of using FoodAPS, and ideas for making future iterations more powerful. Other ERS data sources may also be discussed.
  - An update from Westat on FoodAPS-2 progress
  - **Laurie May** (collection and survey protocols/methods) and **Tom Krenzke** (mathematical/statistics side)
  - User feedback from researchers using FoodAPS-1
  - **Parke Wilde** and **Mehreen Ismail,** Tufts University (data needs for measuring SNAP/non-SNAP differences in food spending or other outcomes, as a representative-use case for thinking about data requirements for FoodAPS and other federal data sources).
  - **Robert Moffitt,** Johns Hopkins (applied research on program outcomes—food expenditure, reporting errors, SNAP purchases impacts).
  - Use of USDA consumer food data system data for health research. Using the Healthy Eating Index to assess the diet quality of the food supply chain
  - **Susan Krebs-Smith,** National Cancer Institute
  - Food and Nutrition Service (FNS)—How does FNS use the information put out by CFDS, and for what purpose?
  - **Melissa Abelev,** FNS
- Panel questions and comments (Bruce Meyer, Eric Rimm, Tim Beatty, Jim Ziliak, Craig Gundersen); open discussion

3:00 Discussion of Meeting #3 content options

3:30 *Adjourn*

Appendix C

Summary, Third Meeting, September 21, 2018

The panel's third meeting, held September 20-21, was intended to broaden the information-gathering phase of the study to include the broader research community that puts Economic Research Service (ERS) data to use. **Colleen Heflin** of Syracuse University, **Justine Hastings** of Brown University, and **Chuck Courtemanche** of Georgia State University presented ideas for improving food and nutrition data—including integration of commercial and administrative data—to inform key policy issues. Among the topics they discussed were the value (and limits) of linking Supplemental Nutrition Assistance Program (SNAP) administrative data with other types of administrative data, such as unemployment insurance (U/I), Medicaid, and K–12 education; the limits of existing survey data; use of retail panel loyalty card data and Rhode Island state administrative records (housed in a secure facility at Brown University) to analyze how SNAP benefits are spent; evidence needed to design a "smarter SNAP"; and food consumption data needs for obesity and other health research.

Amy O'Hara (panel member), **Rachel Shattuck** and **John Eltinge** of the Census Bureau, and **Lisa Mirel** of the National Center for Health Statistics (NCHS) gave presentations on the potential of data integration, linkages for policy research, and the use of administrative data. Practices being developed by the statistical agencies for combining data sources were also discussed, including the Next Generation Data Platform—a collaboration between Census, ERS, and the Food and Nutrition Service (FNS) that links SNAP data (in 19 states and in 39 counties in California) and the Special Supplemental Nutrition Program for Women, Infants, and Children (WIC) data (in 11 states) to Census survey and administrative data.

Rob Santos of the Urban Institute, who is a member of the Feeding America Technical Advisory Group, discussed the collaboration with the Urban Institute on a research program that attempts to detail the frequency of visits to food pantries by individuals, either as a temporary, emergency food source or as a regular supplemental food source. **Alessandro Bonanno** of Colorado State University discussed possible improvements to geospatial information in ERS's food data system (e.g., for assessing the role of the accessibility of food outlets in SNAP participation and effectiveness).

A final open session was held on the use of proprietary data for food policy research. **Mary Muth** of RTI discussed types, sources, and considerations in using store scanner data, household scanner data, and nutrition data from labels for food policy research. **Helen Jensen** of Iowa State described the use of proprietary (scanner) data for understanding issues related to the WIC program. **Carma Hogue** of the U.S. Census Bureau described Census's work on improving economic statistics through web scraping and machine learning to discover, collect, and process data from the web.

C.1. UPDATE ON RECENT DEVELOPMENTS AT ERS AND WITH FOODAPS-2

After a brief welcome from panel chair **Marianne Bitler**, **Jay Variyam**, division director at ERS, updated the panel on three significant developments at ERS:

1. The USDA secretary has proposed realigning ERS with USDA's Office of the Chief Economist—the ERS administrator would report directly to the chief economist instead of the undersecretary for research, education, and economics, as is the current practice.
2. The USDA secretary also proposed relocating ERS functions, along with the National Institute of Food and Agriculture (NIFA), to a new, as-yet undisclosed or unselected location; the target date for relocation is the end of FY 2019. The relocation has implications for the operational side of the Consumer Food Data Program; for example, staffing will potentially be split between two locations, as a few dozen ERS staffers would remain in Washington, DC, while up to 300 others would move. Work with other federal partners, who will be based in Washington, DC, as well as the way ERS handles stakeholder interactions, would by necessity change.
3. In light of new USDA program and policy priorities, ERS has paused FoodAPS-2 implementation. It is assessing the situation and, in the meantime, working with the contractor, Westat, to create a fully functional data collection app.

Mark Denbaly, deputy director for food economics data at ERS, noted that the above changes mean the panel's role in helping ERS is even more important than before, because ERS needs a roadmap from experts in order to prioritize investments. Variyam pointed out that how ERS structures its staff after relocation will affect stakeholder interactions and other interagency activities, in particular the administrative data program, which requires close interaction with agencies within USDA and outside of it. Panel member **Dianne Schanzenbach** stated her concern that critical administrative data products produced in conjunction with other federal agencies, specifically with the Census Bureau, will be impacted if ERS staff relocate. Variyam and Denbaly did not speculate on what those impacts might be and stressed that the roadmap they seek from the panel will be key for the future of the Consumer Food Data Program.

C.2. IMPROVING DATA FOR POLICY RESEARCH

Colleen Heflin of Syracuse University began the session by talking about the role and value of administrative data as it relates to USDA data collection. In comparison to survey data, administrative data

- help minimize the measurement error often found in the self-reporting of program participation;
- can be used to observe monthly benefit receipts to learn about participation dynamics and intensity of participation; and
- provide opportunities to learn about multiple-program participation (e.g., SNAP alone versus SNAP plus Medicaid or SNAP plus the Temporary Assistance for Needy Families [TANF]).

Heflin offered examples of combining SNAP data with three different domains of administrative data: Medicaid, U/I, and education.

Medicaid claims data offer rich information about diagnosis, the date a claim was made, in what setting it was made (emergency room, a hospitalization, a nursing home, a pharmacy), and the cost of a claim. Heflin noted a study (Basu et al., 2017) that looked at hospital admissions for hypoglycemia for low-income patients that occurred during the last week of each month when SNAP benefits may have been exhausted. Linking health data to data from food and nutrition programs can inform researchers about the return on investment of these food and nutrition programs.

Linking SNAP data with U/I data allows researchers to understand the dynamics of the relationship between SNAP participation and work. Specifically, one can observe employment behavior before a household goes on SNAP, what that household earns while it participates in SNAP, and changes that occur in times of transition, that is, what happens to wages preceding SNAP participation and what occurs after participation is completed. Since this can be done by industry, one can get a sense of which industries have employees who participate in SNAP more than others. Looking closer, one can see which people exhaust U/I and then participate in SNAP, or whether they participate in both programs together.

Linking SNAP data with K–12 data—which includes academic performance, attendance, disability services utilized, suspensions, retention, graduation, participation in school meals, etc.—can offer insights into how the timing of participation in SNAP affects educational achievement and health. Participation in school meals programs is supposed to improve academic achievement, but without detailed education data outcomes cannot be observed. As education data include both SNAP and non-SNAP participants, one can observe differences in attainment among those groups.

Heflin noted that the limitation of administrative data in relation to survey data decline when data are linked across programs. Administrative data from SNAP only include participants, but linking the types of datasets mentioned above to SNAP administrative records allows for more coverage of the total population, undermining a key limitation of most administrative data. When SNAP participation dynamics and benefit amounts data are linked to health care claims, U/I, and education data, observations about other people in the household can be made. Thus, the limitation of a single administrative dataset is minimized by adding many more administrative datasets. Heflin stated that more of this should be done. Participation in SNAP and other food and nutrition programs may impact many other domains, such as interactions with the criminal justice system, wage records, health, and education. Survey data on these domains might not be trustworthy or representative, Heflin noted, which speaks to the value of more administrative record linking. Heflin emphasized that much of these data are housed at the state level, as is the case with SNAP. Getting a state to cooperate with research efforts is fraught with challenges. For example:

- Creating data that are useful for researchers is costly for the state, both in the skill required to produce it and in associated opportunity costs.
- Data for a single program are often in multiple files (i.e., there is a demographic file, an eligibility file, and a benefit file), and these files may not have the same timeframe.
- To preserve confidentiality, unique IDs for participants must be created by the state that are not identifiable to researchers.
- Research using state records may result in negative findings—an Urban Institute report (Mills et al., 2014) prepared for ERS found that in some states up to one in four SNAP clients experienced gaps in their food stamp benefits even though they were eligible. While they may be painful for some states to acknowledge, these types

of findings can have positive effects as state administrators and legislators become aware of problems.

Approaching a state to cooperate in a research project can present more challenges, as there are no national standards. Heflin noted that occasionally a researcher may have to meet with an institutional review board before a project is approved, but this varies by state. Data agreements are legal arrangements, so a researcher working at a university will have to involve that university's lawyers, who are often not experts in data agreements. This can cause delays as lawyers are brought up to speed; states may also push back against individual components of a project. When a project is completed, states often stipulate that the researcher destroy the data. While this is a reasonable request for data privacy concerns, it also means that researchers cannot later add to that data, precluding any longitudinal analysis. States may also require that the resulting analysis be reviewed or approved by the state prior to dissemination, although this has not been an issue for Heflin—she has received useful comments or added context from the state that improved the final product.

If a researcher is attempting to link data across multiple agencies, each agency will have its own process: sometimes its own set of lawyers, its own institutional review board, its own data agreement language, and its own linking and de-identification procedures, which then need to be harmonized. This process gets multiplied at each addition of datasets. Finally, in many states refreshing the data means starting the data agreement process again—and since state actors frequently change, this may mean there will be no institutional knowledge of the previous work. Some state officials may remember the researcher from work completed years earlier, but often researchers must start afresh in explaining how the process worked the last time. All of this results in high costs to researchers to use state administrative data. The costs may be summarized this way:

- time to get access (which can take months to years);
- the enormous size of files (costing storage and computational space);
- the requirement to have special skill sets (not just standard survey analysis);
- lack of available codebooks;
- the need to correct a large amount of error in the data; and
- the many differences among the states, as well as each agency within a state sometimes having its own process.

Heflin believes that, nevertheless, these costs of obtaining administrative data are worth the investment, especially as survey responses rates continue to decline and costs associated with surveys rise. These administrative data can produce longitudinal datasets to answer policy questions, for example, tracking investments made in early childhood and their educational outcomes. Once agreements can be reached with states, data become available to researchers in a timely fashion—another advantage over traditional surveys.

Heflin ended by offering six suggestions for improving access to administrative data:

1. Encourage states to make data available to researchers for evaluative purposes when proper data safeguards are in place.
2. Create data agreement standards.
3. Establish 5-year minimum agreements; preferably with clauses that do not require the destruction of data.
4. Make money available to underwrite the state costs (including data analytics training for staff).
5. Make money available to academic researchers to use administrative data for policy-relevant purposes.
6. Formally encourage states to collaborate with researchers to use their data to evaluate state policies and practices.

Justine Hastings of Brown University and Research Improving People's Lives (RIPL) talked about her work combining SNAP data with grocery store scanner data in Rhode Island. This work is underpinned by a customized database created by RIPL that combined all administrative records in the state of Rhode Island for 20 years with detailed information on program participation. Algorithms were developed for identifying individuals across these records, and the data were then anonymized. The records are updated quarterly to keep the database current, something made possible due to the buy-in of state officials to allow access to the records. RIPL gained their confidence by employing robust security procedures—most data they hold are encrypted. If a researcher needs to unencrypt a piece of personally identifiable information, doing so requires a two-party password that sends automated, tamper-proof logs so that every senior team member knows exactly what was done, and when, with that file.

Hastings and state officials sought to understand how SNAP benefits are spent and whether changes in how they are distributed might help the program better meet people's needs; to accomplish this, Rhode Island allowed RIPL access to state SNAP data. Other data Hastings' team utilized were scanner data from a major grocery retailer, USDA FoodAPS data, as well as Nielsen Homescan data—these last two elements were used to see whether the grocery panelists were substantially different or similar to SNAP beneficiaries as a whole.

The store scanner data include loyalty card purchases from February 2006 to December 2012 made in five states by households that shop at the chain at least every other month; this resulted in identifying 486,570 households through 608 million purchase occasions. Each purchase included the following information: main payment method used, characteristics of each product purchased (including product size and weight, text description, and location within taxonomy), and coupon redemption and offers.

Using identification strategies afforded by Rhode Island state participation data, Hastings' team sought to use changes in SNAP enrollment to measure the causal impact of SNAP on food expenditure, such as what is the marginal propensity to consume food (MPCF) using a dollar of SNAP versus a dollar of cash, and to attempt to understand how SNAP enrollment changes measures of shopping effort, which they obtain from their grocery retailer data. They define shopping effort as coupon clipping (when coupons are available), and whether the purchase was for a store brand (i.e., purchase of a cheaper store brand or a more expensive national brand). To account for nutrition, the researchers have built a database to generate several measures of nutrition.

Hastings found (Hastings and Shapiro, 2018) that the MCPF out of SNAP benefits is 0.5 to 0.6 while the MPCF out of cash is much smaller; non-food purchases were not affected. Changes in gasoline prices affected disposable income but did not have an outsized impact on food spending. Hastings also found a small decrease in coupon redemption (shopping effort) and a decrease in the share of store brands purchased, but, again, not in non-food categories.

Hastings noted that these findings are consistent with a model of mental accounting where people feel food-wealthy when they receive a SNAP payment in one sum, and this was reinforced in responses from participants in interviews her team conducted.

Chuck Courtemarche of Georgia State began his remarks by echoing the challenges Colleen Heflin reported earlier: getting data from states can take a very long time. In reference to one of his studies, he noted that it took nearly 2 years for the state to start supplying data and that this occurred only after USDA officials interceded.

Courtemarche then discussed a recent paper (Courtemanche, Denteh, and Tchernis, 2019) about the impacts of SNAP participation on food insecurity, obesity, and food purchases. The motivation for the paper was to look at whether SNAP achieves its goal of improving food security, and whether that goal has unintended consequences. He noted that recent research on causal effects generally finds that SNAP participation reduces food insecurity (Hoynes and Schanzenbach, 2015), but evidence of the causal effect of SNAP participation on obesity is mixed (Gundersen, 2015).

Courtemarche looked at the less-studied phenomenon of measurement error in administrative data using data from FoodAPS. FoodAPS, he noted, offers a unique opportunity to examine misreporting and its consequences, since it contains both self-reported and administrative participation measures.

He and his team went into the study thinking the administrative data would be the accurate, "gold standard" benchmark by which they could examine the extent, causes, and consequences of errors in self-reported participation in SNAP. The availability of two different administrative measures (totals the state provides and totals that could be linked through EBT purchases, discussed below) that did not match one another led Courtemarche's team to undertake a sensitivity analysis to get at the inconsistencies. Their research question changed to: How sensitive are misreporting rates and regression estimates to the use of different coding rules for each of the two administrative measures separately, and to different coding rules for combining the two administrative measures in addition to the self-report rate into a single "true" participation variable? This analysis did not meaningfully affect their initial conclusions. The composition of self-report data from the FoodAPS survey in addition to the two administrative datasets is noted below:

Data characteristics provided by FoodAPS are as follows:

- a nationally representative survey of U.S. households to collect comprehensive data about household food purchases as well as health and nutrition outcomes;
- 4,826 households (SNAP, nonparticipating low-income, and higher income);
- Courtemarche's sample included 2,108 households with income under 250 percent of the federal poverty level, with no missing data for outcomes and controls;
- outcome variables—indicators for food insecurity, very low food security, Healthy Eating Index score, body mass index (BMI), indicators for overweight/obesity, obesity (BMI ≥ 30, severe obesity (BMI ≥ 35); and
- covariates—self-reported SNAP participation and two administrative measures; gender, race, marital status, household size, income, education, age, work, rural tract, and WIC participation.

Data characteristics provided by state administrative data include

- state caseload information from March to November 2012 (not quite a match to survey dates of April 2012 to January 2013);
- variation in quality of data across states (e.g., monthly versus non-monthly data, disbursement date availability, period of caseload data); two states did not report disbursement dates, five did not provide caseload data at all; and
- probabilistic matching of all respondents to SNAP caseload data—based on first name, last name, phone number, house address, and

"certain" matches identified by matching score being above predetermined level.

Data characteristics provided by Electronic Benefits Transfer (EBT) swipes and linkage techniques:

- the state, store ID, EBT account number, date/time of event from April to December 2012;
- deterministic matching—for households matched to caseload data using a known case IDs: only possible in 13 states where ID numbers are the same;
- probabilistic matching—for other households, and a probabilistic match based on store ID, amount, and date; in order for matching to occur, the household had to have a purchase during the survey week; if participants stockpiled food the week before or already ran out of benefits, they would not be captured; and
- no match attempted—if respondent did not self-report either SNAP receipt or any EBT-type payments; thus, they would miss true participants who misreported both of these activities.

Courtemarche concluded that while the FoodAPS' administrative SNAP measures are not perfect, they are adequate, especially when compared to state data. Whatever error there might be does not seem to meaningfully affect conclusions. There is a low false-negative rate, which might be due to the presence of the administrative measures. Having three different measures, two of which are administrative, allows for a combined measure that is probably of a high quality. But the biggest drawback, Courtemarche believes, is missing data. He conceded that it would be better to have administrative measures of participation for other programs like WIC or Medicaid to improve matching.

The major drawback of this analysis is the lack of "causal" research questions that can be answered with FoodAPS. With less than 5,000 households in FoodAPS, it is hard to use inherently inefficient estimators like instrumental variables or regression discontinuity. The lack of time-series variation prevents difference-in-difference or fixed-effects models as well. FoodAPS-2 could be of great value if it allowed for repeated cross-sections, for example, so one could study effects of state- or county-level variables. If there were a way to track even a subset of households over time, Courtemarche thought, that would be a useful improvement.

During open discussion, panel member **Michael Link** asked the three presenters to consider the quality of matching administrative records. He pointed out that there is reasonable agreement on what quality survey methodology is, but the linkages as described by the three panelists are less well-defined. Link also wanted to know whether states that hold these vast administrative datasets have realized their value and started creating their own linkages or have been more open to allowing access from researchers.

Colleen Heflin noted that it varies by state; some are more "enlightened" users than others and have begun their own linkages or allowed more access to researchers, but expertise and resource constraints often hold them back. Justine Hastings noted that a state or any other government entity would need the appropriate technical expertise not only to build the data infrastructure but also to use it. She thinks outside groups are better equipped to provide these services to states and to actually offer them the analyses they want and need. **Courtemarche** agreed that there must be incentives for both data providers and researchers to work together if we are to see real progress.

Panel member **Diane Schanzenbach** asked Hastings how the research community, including USDA, can obtain more and higher-quality data, whether these data are bought from private companies or obtained from government sources. Schanzenbach also asked for thoughts on how well separating or combining these multiple data sources represent actual spending patterns. Hastings pointed out that data from food pantries, soup kitchens, and from credit card purchases for food could enrich what is known about consumption thus informing spending. Credit card data would also be valuable in determining food-away-from-home purchases. Hasting thought survey data are useful, but the recall limitations of respondents as well as declining response rates is of concern to her.

C.3. DATA INTEGRATION AND LINKAGES FOR POLICY RESEARCH USING ADMINISTRATIVE DATA

Panel member **Amy O'Hara** began the session by describing the international set of best practices for the handling of sensitive data, especially the use of administrative data or health data. Key to this handling are the five "safes": safe projects, safe people, safe settings, safe data, and safe outputs—the federal statistical system, as a whole, performs these functions well. The system has infrastructure in place so that the linkages described by earlier presenters can be done with the lowest risk possible.

Knowing why data are collected is another component. Are they being collected to answer questions pertinent to an agency or for Congressional oversight? Knowing who developed the collection, who approved it, and how much latitude the people that are conducting the collection and analysis are also valuable in determining whether data are fit for research purposes. Researchers must also consider how the data are handled, particularly when attempting linkages. Using linked, harmonized data relies on the data providers curating their data for such purposes. Any breaks in either collection or treatment will affect linkages.

O'Hara pointed out that such curation has occurred at agencies such as NCHS, the Census Bureau, and some local governments, but access to these data can be limited to employees of the agency and certain academics who can navigate the process to make use of these, often, sensitive data. The Census Bureau has established policies for interested parties to gain access. The point is, O'Hara continued, that providers must have confidence that a data user would handle the data responsibly. Further, the location of any data analysis also affects access. Questions that must be answered include

- Where will the work be done? Is it going to be at the Census Bureau? Is it going to be at the headquarters of the private company?
- Will the researcher be furnished the data via a laptop?
- Will the researcher have to go to a data enclave? This could be a federal research data center, an enclave administered by a third party, such as the National Opinion Research Center, or an enclave maintained by a state—Washington State and South Carolina have such enclaves.

Another best practice O'Hara mentioned for the handling of sensitive data concerns the output data and its quality. Research papers or dashboards may have to be reviewed prior to dissemination at least to ensure the correct privacy protections are being applied so that those individuals in the data cannot be re-identified and that they have consented to the new analysis being conducted. O'Hara noted that the Census Bureau's surveys no longer ask individuals for consent for linkage because the data will be used only for statistical purposes when they are linked. The cost of standing up and maintaining a linkage operation is usually substantial, especially if one is interested in doing time-series analyses. With respect to output quality, O'Hara said that one has to be particularly interested in coverage. For example, the Longitudinal Employer-Household Dynamics Program (LEHD) program at the Census Bureau has data from only 13 states. While this may be sufficient for Census's purposes, it may not be sufficient to answer broader policy questions such as levels of food security.

Rachel Shattuck of the Census Bureau described work being done at the bureau in estimating SNAP and WIC eligibility and participation. Congress authorizes the bureau to collect administrative records to improve survey operations. Examples include

- researching and developing applications of administrative records for use in Census and survey operations including imputation, evaluating coverage, and sampling frame improvement;

- conducting innovative social scientific academic research using linked data to improve estimates about characteristics and behavior of the U.S. population; and
- linking multiple data sources to create new statistical products, for example, SNAP and WIC program eligibility and participation estimates.

An aspect of the Census Bureau's partnership with USDA that is of note for the panel is linking administrative and survey data to understand and improve models of SNAP eligibility and participation rates. These linked data can also benefit states in that they gain information about participants and eligible nonparticipants as well as for outreach to prospective participants—24 states have agreements with the Bureau to share their SNAP data, while 11 states have a similar agreement to share WIC data.

The Census Bureau acquires administrative records via legal agreements with states and the data are encrypted when transmitted. When the files arrive at the Census Bureau they are placed on a secure, isolated server where a very small number of staff who have authorization to see these data create matching identifiers and remove all personally identifiable information (PII).The data then become available to researchers for use. Access to the data requires producing a proposal that describes data use, research question, and methods, etc. In some cases the agency that owns the data may need to review the output before submission for publication can occur. The final step performed at the Bureau is linkage of the administrative records with existing survey data.

For SNAP and WIC linking, Shattuck continued, states are requested to provide: participant PII such as name, date of birth and Social Security number (SSN), as well as address history, eligibility certification, and termination dates, and monthly history of benefits received. To link data, the Census Bureau uses the Person Validation System, which uses the PII and a probabilistic matching technique to assign a unique identifier called a Protected Identification Key (PIK). Address information is also used to generate a unique address identifier. Shattuck reiterated that before researchers can use the data, PII is removed, and what remains on the file is a unique identifier that also appears in survey data. The Bureau can then match the same individuals who appear in the administrative records to respondents in the survey data.

Specifically, for SNAP and WIC data, sources and estimation method involve

- *Modeling for eligibility*. Data from the American Community Survey (ACS) that includes annual individual-level microdata with a reference period of 12 months prior to survey month. Those who can be modeled-eligible for SNAP are individuals in families with annual income below the FNS eligibility threshold. For WIC, the modeled-eligible include children under age 4 years who are on Medicaid, or receiving SNAP or TANF (this is self-reported), and an annual family income below the FNS eligibility threshold. The Bureau cannot measure pregnancy with ACS data, so pregnant women are excluded from eligibility estimates.

- *Linkage of ACS sample records to administrative records to identify participation.* For SNAP, this includes individuals of all ages, while for WIC it is children ages 0-4 years, and women ages 15 years and older.
- *Aggregation and calculation of coverage rates and distributions of characteristics at state and county level.* This is done to create table packages and data visualizations, which are sent to states after being cleared for disclosure avoidance.

Estimates provided by the Bureau to states generally include more information about participants—such as sub-state eligibility and coverage rates that are often stratified by demographic and economic characteristics, and by county—than the states can collect on their own. The Bureau can also estimate an eligible nonparticipating population that include characteristics—this can be helpful with outreach to eligible people who are not participating.

The Bureau faces challenges in producing these estimates. In particular, full state and territory participation is hindered by high rates of turnover in state agencies and limited resources. Some states might want to give their data to the Bureau but they may have limited technical ability for how to do so. Some states are reluctant to share their data because they have concerns about confidentiality, while some are concerned that their data will be made public and they may be compared unfavorably to other states.

Speaking about data quality, Shattuck said the Bureau tries to make it as easy as possible for states to share their data with them, emphasizing the basic information that they need from states to create a unique identifier and the basic information needed to model participation. They tend to get what they need to create table packages, but other data on the file may vary from state to state that affects usability. While administrative records are not representative of the U.S. population, they can have information on hard to count populations, such as low-income children who do not appear in the decennial census. The Bureau has newly created a data quality branch that helps with technical issues, while program staff are tasked with verifying that files can be accessed, generating SAS datasets, producing documentation, and utilizing multiple analysts for quality assurance. Shattuck mentioned next steps in data quality at the Bureau, which include more research on where data quality issues typically occur and how they can be anticipated and addressed, more automation of the quality control process, and better standardization of variables and documentation across states.

John Eltinge, Census Bureau, spoke about data quality issues when integrating multiple data sources from the perspective of the Federal Committee on Statistical Methodology of the Washington Statistical Society, of which he is a member.

The first, *inferential* quality, involves having a clear vision when communicating what an estimate encompasses in a given setting, and the related inferential goals or questions one is trying to address with respect to those estimates. Transparency of methods and processes is required, especially the level of aggregation (e.g., geography), the quality of the information at the specified level of aggregation, the extent of stakeholder risk incurred through poor quality or break in series, as well as conveying the value of transparency of the above concepts. It may be challenging, Eltinge continued, to convey the importance of inferential quality to technical specialists, "power users," the media, and general public—the last two groups especially so—but it should be attempted nonetheless.

Discussing quality of *data sources*, Eltinge sees a need to allocate resources to ensure satisfactory balance of multiple dimensions of quality, risk, and cost—all elements that affect the design of any data collection and analysis. Methodology will also have to be improved to create an extension of standard total survey error models to integration of multiple sources, especially in relation to population coverage and missing variables. Practically speaking, taking action on the above items would involve finding better data sources, such as more administrative records or bridge surveys, and making inferences about current sources and accounting for errors.

The risks to data quality involve the loss of, or major changes in, data sources—this is well known to any researcher or analyst. Changes in a production system and the related costs, as well as disclosure, are other factors. These issues also need to be addressed through tools designed to identify and manage risk. Below the federal level there are implications for management and integration of regional data sources, especially the costs incurred in linking datasets. These costs borne by agencies and researchers can be substantial, so they must be included in budgets

Eltinge concluded that in the "old world" when sample surveys were a dominant mode of data collection, there was a high degree of control over nearly everything that took place in data collection, analysis, and inference, but this is not the case when linking multiple data sources that include administrative records.

In the discussion that followed this session, panel member **Jim Ziliak** asked whether states had asked explicitly for data products or other resources when sharing their data with the Census Bureau. **Amy O'Hara** said that, in her experience at the Bureau, if states asked for money to defray reasonable costs, the Bureau paid. John Eltinge pointed out that some states and smaller geographical units are keen to acquire economic measures about their locale, but these often very small units do not have enough observations in data to be released in full. The recent Bureau notion of a "privacy budget" in disclosure limitation influences how much local-area data can be released.

Panel member **Craig Gundersen** asked about the varying level of competence in data science in states and whether they might want an expert to help them organize their data in more effective ways to produce more useful products for both the state and federal partners. He also asked whether states were imposing higher restrictions on federal partners, in terms of confidentiality, than the states themselves are imposing. Chuck Courtemanche thought aligning incentives and giving states something of value—a specific data product—is important because many states do not consider the output of researchers, by itself, to be a worthwhile investment. He noted that the disposition of an individual official at a state can greatly affect that state's cooperation; showing that person how the research will benefit their office or agency can be helpful.

In terms of confidentiality, from a federal perspective, Eltinge pointed out that federal requirements vary by agency and type of data handled (health, tax, education, etc.). He thought the implementation of a privacy budget approach to assess what the incremental risk of disclosure is regardless of what other entities, including states, do would be a fundamental change.

Cordell Golden, NCHS, described a data linkage project his unit is currently undertaking using information from Department of Housing and Urban Development (HUD) Rental Assistance programs.

The motivation for the linkage lies in the strategic goals of both NCHS and HUD, results of the Foundations for Evidence-Based Policymaking Act, and several directives on the use of administrative records issued by the U.S. Office of Management and Budget (OMB) of the Executive Office of the President.

These three rental assistance programs to which NCHS has linked data are (i) Public Housing (PH), which is federally funded and regulated but managed by local housing authorities, (ii) Housing Choice Voucher (HCV), which is HUD's largest rental assistance program for monthly rental assistance payment to assist very low income families, and (iii) Multifamily (MF), where there is a contract between HUD and owners of a development.

NCHS views its partnership with HUD to be mutually beneficial, where both agencies bring some level of expertise to the table. NCHS has experts in health and data linkages—the Special Projects Branch is the data linkage program at NCHS. HUD brings experts on housing dynamics.

A memorandum of understanding was signed in which NCHS would perform the linkage and would also waive the federal statistical research data center (FSRDC) fees for researchers from HUD that would use the data. HUD would be tasked with providing geocoding services for the NCHS surveys that were to be linked. Two NCHS surveys used in the linkage project were the National Health Interview Survey (NHIS) and the National Health and Nutrition Examination Survey (NHANES).

Augmenting the survey data with longitudinal administrative data facilitates richer analysis and allows NCHS to address questions that cannot be addressed with survey data alone. It also enhances the administrative data by adding socio-demographics, health behaviors, and other outcomes from the survey. The linkage criteria are as follows: the respondent must

- provide sufficient personally identifying information (SSN, name, date of birth, sex);
- not explicitly refuse linkage; and
- not refuse to answer question about public housing (NHIS-only).

For child respondents, only information gathered prior to their 18th birthday may be linked due to consent rules. NCHS follows a deterministic approach and uses SSN, date of birth, sex, and name as identifier.

NCHS has produced several reports based on these linkages. One such report describes the methodology for the linkage.[1] Although this report was produced by NCHS, it was done in collaboration with HUD, particularly on issues related to the guidelines on how the data should be analyzed. Other examples of NCHS research include "Housing Assistance and Blood Lead Levels: Children in the United States, 2005–2012A" and "HUD Housing Assistance Associated with Lower Uninsurance Rates and Unmet Medical Need," which examines whether receiving HUD housing assistance is associated with improved access to health care. Many reports have also been produced by HUD that describe adults and children who receive HUD benefits.[2]

Access to the linked data is similar to accessing Census Bureau data described by Rachel Shattuck. NCHS has research data centers in Atlanta and Washington, DC, and they are affiliated with FSRDCs around the country as well. Research proposals are required but NCHS has feasibility files on its website that provide an indicator on eligibility status, whether or not the survey participant was eligible to be included in the linkage, and whether the participant provided consent. The files also tell researchers whether NCHS found the respondent in a HUD program. These files are designed for researchers, as they prepare their FSRDC proposal, to estimate their maximum analytic sample.

---

[1] See https://www.cdc.gov/nchs/data/series/sr_01/sr01_060.pdf.

[2] See https://www.huduser.gov/portal/publications/Health-Picture-of-HUD.html and https://www.huduser.gov/portal/publications/Health-Picture-of-HUD-Assisted-Children.html.

Golden concluded by noting that the linkage project with HUD demonstrates an effective collaboration between two federal agencies, which both agencies plan to continue to produce this rich data source.

C.4. ADDITIONAL NONGOVERNMENTAL SOURCES FOR FILLING DATA GAPS IN ERS'S CONSUMER FOOD DATA SYSTEM PROGRAM

Rob Santos, The Urban Institute, spoke about projects and reports coming out of Feeding America's (FA) flagship survey, *Hunger in America* (HIA).[3] As background, Santos noted that Feeding America is a network of 200 independent food banks throughout the country. These food banks partner with more than 60,000 agencies (pantries, meal programs, etc). Annually, they provide service to more than 40 million individuals and give out over 3 million pounds of food nationally.

FA has a robust research group that attempts to answer three principal research questions: who are the clients, what are their needs, and how can we serve them better. To help better identify their clients, FA has an ongoing effort to track client data, registering every distinct individual and then tracking them over time, including how often they go to the food bank, what do they get, and so forth. The client portrait can identify specific vulnerable subgroups to determine what the group's needs are, with a heavy emphasis on social demographic characteristics. This information is also used during FA fundraising activities to inform funders about the types of clients FA have and are helping. Any changes in distinct client count can be used to assess overall productiveness of FA programs. HIA includes rich data specific to clients, and FA gathers information on food insecurity, nutrition, and any ancillary additional measures such as housing stability, health issues, employment, basic household needs, and food insecurity. Evaluation research in assessing outcomes of FA's clients results in pilot programs. This is done to ensure clients' needs are met as circumstances change.

HIA is the largest study of charitable feeding in the country with 63,000 interviewed participants using Audio-CASI (in the most recent version). It is done in all participating food banks on a quadrennial basis. The design involves total probability sampling, sample surveys, multistage sampling, and clustered design—about 16,000 agencies are sampled to get the 60,000 completed interviews. The size and scope allows FA to have a micro-database with different types of characteristics allowing deep dives into small subgroups such as seniors or veterans. It provides valid national statistical estimates, and at the food bank level.

---

[3] See https://www.feedingamerica.org/hunger-in-america.

Disadvantages of HIA include the cost of the survey—about $10 million, which includes food banks providing staff to help coordinate the sampling and the interviewing operation the field—and its periodicity of being done once every 4 years. Santos noted that results that are 4 years old may not represent the population, especially during a time of economic upheaval. There is a desire for more contemporaneous data to enable rapid interventions and to collect information about hot topics of the day. This desire to be more nimble and contemporary has led to redesign attempts to lower the cost of the survey. An ACS-style rolling survey of 5,000 respondents a year was discussed, but operation costs only decreased slightly while burden on food bank staff was still high.

Another attempt to redesign HIA is under way. Since the gold standard, 60,000 respondent survey is untenable from a budget perspective, FA is reducing the scope. Statistical national estimates will not be available but suggestive insights—Santos's terminology—would still be useful. FA would not be able to say nationally that X percent of clients belong to this ethnic or age group, with a margin of error, but it might acquire enough information to make decisions. Making the collection a data analytics operation is the first step. This involves creating a taxonomy of food banks that sorts them using analytic approaches and the information FA has on food banks and clients to create 12 to 20 groups, and then selecting about 10 percent of them for further analysis. The results might look like a surveillance type operation. Data could be analyzed and combined for, say, 20 sites to look at the different subgroups. The insights gleamed from the analysis would be suggestive, as opposed to point estimates, of the population. Santos thinks this might be good enough to create strategies and prioritize programs.

Santos concluded by noting that the panel, in its recommendations, has the challenge of operating within the current policy environment, which means smaller budgets and pressure to do more. The new process Santos outlined may be beneficial for the panel in thinking through ways of getting the types of data that ERS needs to make decisions without necessarily making it a point estimate with a margin of error.

Alessandro Bonanno, Colorado State University, provided some thoughts and insights improving geospatial information in ERS's food data system. He started by describing the common metrics that have been used in the analysis of food access: store location, distance traveled, store availability, and pricing. He said that these are related to metrics listed in a systematic review by Crepsi et al. (2012): availability, accessibility, affordability, acceptability, and accommodation. Availability and accessibility are covered in the common metrics. Affordability deals with prices. He noted that few studies have looked at either the combined cost of food and time to get to the store or food price differentials. Acceptability is typically measured in consumer surveys of consumer perceptions about a store. Accommodation is not really being focused on in research.

Bonanno's first research question was whether access to food stores affects a household's decision to participate in SNAP. Bonanno said that he does not think this question has been addressed as yet. Another research question, he said, is whether the effectiveness of SNAP benefits is affected by access to food stores. A number of researchers have used ERS products to answer this question. For example, researchers have used FoodAPS to look at the facts of the SNAP food cycle, whether participants "stretch" benefits by shopping at cheaper stores, how SNAP benefits affect healthfulness of diet, and the relationship between food security, SNAP participation and the food environment (a new project under way at Colorado State University).

He described the ERS *Food Access Research Atlas* (FARA) as a product that is very useful in assessing some issues of food access at the census tract and county levels. It does not provide geocoded data, but instead provides aggregate data at the census tract level. Tracts are marked as being low-income or not, and low-food-access or not. Indicators include vehicle access, households with limited access (by number of children and mile radius). Previous versions also included a food desert indicator.

FARA is currently available for 2015 (the previous version was 2010). However, the methods have changed across the years, and though they are well documented, the differences between the 2010 and 2015 versions make analysis over time difficult. Having regularly updated versions of FARA would benefit researchers.

Bonanno said that he thinks that FoodAPS is the one dataset that allows researchers to best understand the environment that low-income households are exposed to. It has the largest amount of information to help answer questions about food insecurity, SNAP participation, and how SNAP benefits are used along with information on store location and distance traveled to stores. FoodAPS includes the geocoded location where the food acquisition event took place, including whether it was a SNAP authorized store, and the geocodes (latitude and longitude) of the household, so that distances between store of purchase and home can be calculated, and are also part of the data record. FoodAPS includes an indicator as to whether the tract is a low-access area and whether household has vehicle access.

Bonanno described research questions as a way to motivate a discussion of data needs. The simplistic question was, "Does where you shop affect how SNAP benefits are used?"

He noted that the first thing to determine is why a low-income/SNAP household decided to shop (or use their SNAP benefits) at a given food outlet. To properly address this question the following information is needed: geocodes of household and store locations—both where they shopped and locations of alternative stores; number of SNAP-approved stores within driving distance; store characteristics, locations, and prices (to model the household decision); and where shoppers work, commuting routes, and changes in routes across seasons. Observations over time are important to address changes in preference.

Bonanno said that FoodAPS has much of this information, but not all. Data needed for a good analysis of this simple question include a time series of FoodAPS with a detailed geocoded place component; information about shopping habits, and commuting patterns; geocoded information on store location and type provided as a time series (including a record of store openings and closings over time); and summaries of driving distance from home to different stores.

Bonanno stated that enabling researchers to match the many existing restricted use, administrative, and proprietary datasets produced by different agencies and companies might benefit research more than collecting more data. He cited Courtemanche, Denteh, and Tchernis (2019), who linked the Consumer Expenditure Survey, information from the food security supplement (with respondent's location), and Walmart data at an FSRDC.

C.5. USING PROPRIETARY DATA FOR FOOD POLICY RESEARCH

Mary Muth, Research Triangle Institute, described proprietary data: the types, sources, and considerations in using store scanner data, household scanner data, and nutrition data from labels for food policy research. Muth said she has worked with scanner data since about 2000. Originally, such work was done for the Food and Drug Administration (FDA), and more recently with ERS, the USDA's Food Safety and Inspection Service (FSIS), FNS, and the Robert Wood Johnson Foundation. To start, she defined the terminology used for different types of scanner data:

Store scanner data—weekly transactions data provided by retailers

- Includes products with barcodes and random-weight products
- Data obtained by ERS comprise sales data from individual stores or retailer marketing areas and represent an unprojected (unweighted) subset of the total IRI store data

Household scanner data—purchases recorded by a panel of households using an in-home scanner or mobile app

- Includes products with barcodes and, for a portion of the panel, random-weight products
- Data obtained by ERS represent the entire panel, both static households (with weights) and non-static households (without weights)

Nutrition label data—information from labels including calories, nutrient quantities, daily values, serving size, product claims, and (sometimes) ingredient lists

These data are collected for commercial purposes, and are not necessarily designed for research purposes, and data vendors must protect their competitive information and confidentiality of households.

Types of Data and Suppliers

Muth first noted common terminology about scanner data, saying that one hears about Universal Product Codes (UPC), Global Trade Identification Numbers (GTIN), and European Article Numbering (EAN). She noted that the official term is GTIN, but they are commonly called UPCs. She likes to use the term *barcode*, because everybody understands what that means. These terms are all interchangeable in some sense.

Muth then summarized the data suppliers for household and store data and their products. She said that there are three different suppliers of household and store data within the United States and four suppliers worldwide.

- IRI provides household data in its Consumer Network and store data, in InfoScan. It collects data in 10 other countries. They also collect auxiliary data, including the label data.
- Nielson provides household data in Homescan, and they also provide household data in 25 other countries. Nielsen provides store data in Scantrack and also provides store data in 100 other countries. Homescan data are from scanning panels; Nielsen also has household data that is collected through nonscanning panels.
- SPINS has no household data and includes only natural and specialty gourmet stores in the United States.
- Kantar is a big supplier outside of the United States. This is important, because Kantar data are used by many researchers outside the United States.

Muth noted that there is only one consumer panel in the United States, the National Consumer Panel. It is a joint venture by Nielsen and IRI to avoid the duplication inherent in having two different panels operating in the United States. The National Consumer Panel includes about 120,000 households. Both companies use the Consumer Network Panel to prepare their household panel products, but they process the data in different ways. She summarized her analysis of the methodologies used by Nielsen and IRI, explaining differences between the two in how they determine which households to include in the static panel, in price assignment methods, and in procedures for weighting the data to get national totals.

The household data that ERS obtains from IRI represents the entire panel, both static households (those with weights for estimating national estimates) and non-static households (no weights). This has some advantages in terms of being able to look at the differences between the entire panel and those that are not considered reliable enough reporters to be included in the static panel.

The store data that ERS obtains from IRI are a portion of all of the data that IRI collects from stores. They comprise sales data from individual stores or from what IRI calls retailer marketing areas, and make up an unweighted subset of the total IRI dataset. The data that IRI is not providing to ERS are data from smaller stores. IRI considers small store data as extremely proprietary because they are used to produce other IRI data products for their main clients, retailers and food manufacturers.

Muth cautioned that it is important to recognize that companies like IRI and Nielsen put these databases together for their own commercial purposes. They use these data for analysis products to provide to retailers and to manufacturers. The data are not necessarily designed for research purposes. That does not mean the data should not be used, but rather that the user needs to understand the data to best interpret and use them.

Muth described the nutrition label data and its suppliers. Food labels link the barcode with label information such as calories, nutrient, quantities, daily values, serving sizes, and product claims. Sometimes ingredient lists are also available. She identified eight suppliers of label data in the United States, some of whom also collect the data in other countries: FoodSwitch, Gladstone and Nutritionix, IRI, Kentar, Label Insight, Mintel, Nielsen BrandBank, and the USDA Branded Food Products Database (described in Appendix B). Some of suppliers may collect information through apps where consumers scan the barcodes of things that they are consuming, particularly through fitness apps.

Muth said that she recently learned that Gladstone, Label Insight, and Nielsen are offering these data products to retailers to help them optimize location of products on shelves.

Analyzing Scanner Data

Muth described her own experiences in assessing and analyzing scanner data. She said that many years ago, when ERS started working with the Nielsen data, they had the foresight to try to understand more about how the data are collected and what the statistical properties are. As a result, Muth, Siegel, and Zhen (2007) were prepared to assess and document the properties of Nielsen Homescan data. This was important because commercial companies, such as Nielsen, do not necessarily prepare the kind of documentation a researcher needs. Also as part of that effort Zhen and colleagues

(2009) compared weighted expenditures from the Nielsen Homescan data with those from the Consumer Expenditure Survey, documenting possible underreporting in the scanner data. Sweitzer and colleagues (2018) found that the IRI Consumer Network also showed underreporting of food expenses when compared to the Consumer Expenditure Survey and FoodAPS.

Muth said that these studies document the underreporting of purchases recorded by panelists who are asked to scan all purchases. It is clear that not all participating households scan everything they buy. This may be because of the burden of participating on the panel, or there is something else going on to cause this difference.

Muth and colleagues (2013) describe a project in which questions were taken from the Health and Diet Survey and the Flexible Consumer Behavior Survey. A sample was selected from the Consumer Network Panel and asked the same questions. A comparison of responses revealed that the household panelists were more price-conscious, more concerned with taste, less concerned with ease of food preparation, and prepared and ate fewer meals at home. Muth et al. (2017) used information from Homescan and from NHANES to try to better estimate food losses from purchase to consumption for the ERS Loss Adjusted Food Availability System.

For the FDA, Muth and her colleagues developed the models that were used to estimate the costs of the new nutrition facts panel. Underlying the two models for estimating the cost of labeling and the cost of reformulation were the Nielsen Scantrack data. Those models have also been used by other agencies to look at different types of labeling regulations. See Muth et al. (2015a, 2015b).

Muth pointed to her ERS research (Muth et al., 2016) that assessed and documented the IRI Consumer Network, Infoscan, and IRI label data. The information from that report was discussed in the second workshop (see Appendix B). Giombi, Muth, and Levin (2018) compared hedonic models using the nutrition data from the IRI food label database versus Gladstone label data.

Muth said that in collaboration with ERS, she analyzed the differences in reported expenditures between commercial household scanner data and Consumer Expenditure Survey matter in a food demand system. She said a study for FDA that is in review used scanner data to model the impact of health communications on market outcomes. Current work for ERS will use IRI consumer data to update some estimates of consumer-level food loss. Under a RWJF grant she and ERS colleagues are using the IRI data to track the reformulation of foods over time and to simulate the effects of improving nutritional quality of foods commonly purchased by households with children. She is also working on a project for FSIS, in collaboration with ERS, to estimate the cost of updating safe handling instructions on all meat and poultry products.

Muth described the considerations for researchers who use proprietary household, store, and label data. For *household data*, researchers should remember that

- households that participate are likely different from the general population
  - the intensive data collection process is somewhat burdensome
  - participants are possibly more aware or more price-conscious consumers
- some types of households are less likely to meet criteria for inclusion in a static panel
  - For example, in IRI Consumer Network data, younger (under age 35) households, lower income households, Black and Hispanic households, and households with children are less likely to meet static panel criteria
- prices are typically not exact prices paid by the household
  - prices are assigned using store scanner data based on where household shopped
- data are weighted based on demographics, not shipment or expenditure totals

For *Store Data*, researchers should remember that

- Not all stores are represented in the data
  - Data collection process is not designed to capture sales at smaller, independent stores (data may be collected but not available for research)
- Private-label product data (about 18 percent of all food)
  - Not provided by all retailers
  - Aggregation of data by some retailers prevents calculation of unit prices
- Random-weight data (e.g., produce, meat, deli, bakery)
  - Not provided by all stores
  - Product information is fairly limited
- Projection factors (or weights)
  - Not provided to ERS with the data they purchase; therefore unable to calculate representative estimates (possible to obtain weighted totals but not by store)

RTI has a contract to develop weights for use by ERS in which control totals are being calculated using restricted Census Bureau data.

For *Food Label Data,* researchers should remember that

- Tracking products over time is challenging
  - Manufacturers assign new barcodes to existing products when substantial changes occur; therefore, difficult to distinguish new product entrants from existing products with new barcodes
- Label databases are not necessarily updated for all products every year
  - Need to match label data with sales data to ensure active products
- Not all vendors include the ingredient list or include it as one long concatenated field
  - Can require substantial effort to parse ingredient lists
- May require multiple data sources to cover all products of interest
- Data fields will be changing with the roll-out of the new Nutrition Facts Label (e.g., added sugars, vitamin D, potassium)

Muth provided her thoughts on needed future research concerning the various proprietary data sources. The first need is to better understand the differences between households in the static panel versus the entire panel in terms of demographics and differences in knowledge, attitudes, and behaviors. Because IRI provides information on the static and the non-static panel, that analyses can be done now. Second, she said, is the need to better understand the implications of the price assignment methods used by IRI and Nielsen, and particularly how much variation there is across stores and locations in a chain. Third is to understand more about food manufacturer and retailer practices regarding barcode assignments; the assignment of barcodes affects the ability to track changes in the healthiness of the food supply over time. Fourth is to consider improving the coverage of label data by using multiple vendors. Fifth, and finally, is the need to consider how best to use loyalty card data, should it become available. However, loyalty card data should not be considered a replacement for panel data because a household may shop at multiple outlets.

Muth noted that as part of her research she and her colleagues have identified about 150 peer-reviewed publications on food policy research projects using some form of scanner or label data. She thinks that proprietary data will continue to be important for analyzing the effects of changes in federal nutrition programs and changes in the regulations on the healthiness of the food supply, and/or cost benefit analyses of new labeling regulations. They are already being used in local jurisdictions for analyzing effects of local regulations particularly for beverage tax initiates. They could also be useful for analyzing effects of voluntary industry initiatives, such as the convenience store initiative. Two other important applications include looking at the effects of food safety outbreaks on sales and calculating price indices that can be used as a basis for other research studies.

In conclusion, Muth said, despite all the challenges they present, there is really no comparable data source to store-based and household-based scanner data, in terms of the granularity, detail, and frequency, and for much food policy research that needs to be done, there is no alternative data source at all.

Helen Jensen, from Iowa State University, was a member of the panel that authored the 2017 report, *Review of WIC Food Packages: Improving Balance and Choice: Final Report.* The panel used Homescan household panel data as part of this effort. She has also worked on other studies that use scanner data in collaboration with ERS.

Jensen said that for purposes of the WIC analysis, household scanner data were most important. The three main goals of the WIC analysis were, first, to study household purchase behavior; second, to determine prices and price indices for WIC food items; and third, to evaluate the cost of alternative WIC food packages, assess package design, and conduct a regulatory impact analysis. Because of the flexibility of using the Homescan scanner data, Jensen and colleagues were able to evaluate various food package contents meeting food item specifications (types of milk, types of yogurt, etc.), evaluate those items, and talk about the implications for the cost of the program. These analyses contributed to the development of costing for the regulatory impact analysis.

Jensen's research focused on looking at the purchase behavior of WIC participants and WIC-eligible low-income nonparticipant households to examine food selection and choices for at home use. For these population groups, they wanted to determine the share of expenses associated with different types of approved WIC products, such as whole-fat milk versus other milk products. These may be affected by WIC program participation, and the information can be used to evaluate program changes and regional differences over time.

Jensen said that in 2009, states moved to expand the list of whole grain foods that were included in the WIC food packages. The panel used the Homescan household panels that bridged this period, incorporating detailed data by state on the timing of the implementation of the regulations, and looking at the purchase behavior for whole grain products before and after the switch.

First, Jensen commented on representation of the low-income population on Homescan. She showed estimated percentages of the self-reported WIC population in Homescan for several years, both weighted and unweighted. In all years, the unweighted percentages were much lower, indicating that the low-income population is underrepresented in the Homescan panel.

To verify self-reported WIC status, the panel analyzed the household composition, income reporting, and age over time (for those in multiple panel years). They found that among those reporting that they were WIC participants, nearly 40 percent were ineligible according to their analysis.

After the categories of WIC participant and eligible WIC nonparticipant were refined, the panel used pooled 3-year data to estimate expenditures and quantities before and after the package changed. Jensen said that both descriptive statistics and subsequent analysis using propensity score matching and a difference-in-difference approach supported the conclusion that the package change increased the amount of whole grain cereal products that were purchased by the household.

Jensen said that one of the advantages of the scanner data for the purpose of her study was the ability to construct detailed prices for food items with the characteristics that the WIC program was dictating for those items. This was based on searching food label databases and identifying keywords associated with approved products. Store brands were a challenge because they did not have product descriptors. Depending on the state, not all store brands are accepted as WIC food options. With the estimated prices, the panel was able to evaluate the cost of various food package options as part of a regulatory impact analysis.

Jensen summarized the advantages and concerns or challenges they had during their study. First, detailed product descriptions are a key advantage. The timeliness of the data, and the ability to match purchases to the household data for the analysis and evaluation, were all benefits from the store data.

Jensen noted that the first challenge was a concern as to whether the population was representative. Homescan updates household data once a year. As a result, the data have a once-a-year report as to whether or not a household was participating in WIC. The assumption is that WIC expenditures are captured through purchase transactions, but these may not be complete.

Jensen said that there is evidence that most WIC participants use larger retail stores. However, they were uncertain as to what was happening with the WIC formulate, the infant formula. A participant might go to Walmart when they have a car and buy most of their formula, because it is heavy. They might also go to some store that was not participating in the IRI Infoscan. She noted that non-UPC-coded products were not well captured. The data are not complete for purchases of fruit and vegetable components with the WIC case value voucher (CVV). The data would have included a 3-pound bag of apples with a UPC code, but not a purchase of loose apples.

Jensen continued that there are opportunities to link datasets now that did not exist before. Extending those possibilities will improve what can be done with the data. Using the barcode may allow better linkages to some of the state-maintained databases on state-approved products for WIC.

Jensen noted that another panel she worked on (NASEM 2017) was charged with considering science breakthroughs in food and nutrition for 2030. Much of the advancement is projected to be in the food production area. However, it is clear that there are breakthroughs in terms of the types of data that are being generated for the food supply, improvements due to block chain technology and other data technologies in terms of being able to track and identify the flow of products. These will not necessarily impact WIC. But they do offer opportunities for improvements in data and analysis in the long term.

She noted that capturing data in the future may be even more challenging, for example if food is purchased through Amazon and delivered through drones. Finally, Jensen noted that the states are maintaining much more information on foods that are approved and redemption data in electronic form. Developing or maintaining the ability to link to these data through coding may offer future benefits in tracking capabilities.

Carma Hogue, U.S. Census Bureau, described the Census Bureau's work on using web scraping and machine learning to discover, collect, and process data from the web, with a goal to improve economic statistics. First, Hogue provided the big data context and some web-scraping background. She talked about SABLE (a web-scraping software product) and some of its experiences with web scraping.

For the big data context, she said that the economic directorate has been researching alternative data sources and big data methodologies for 4 or 5 years. They are considering quality, costs, and skill sets, whether they have them and what it would take to get them. As background for web scraping she noted that the Census Bureau has many surveys, including surveys of federal, state, and local governments. For some of these entities, much of the data to be collected on surveys is available online. Currently, analysts manually access the data from websites. If Census could develop an automated way to scrape that data, it could reduce respondent and analyst burden.

Hogue said that their definition of web scraping is an automated process of collecting data from an online source. Web crawling is an automated process of systematically visiting and reading web pages.

She described policy issues as well, first the issue of informed consent. Census is currently evaluating a new notice about web-scraping activities that Statistics Canada has just posted. It is also considering *Federal Register* notices; however, they were informed that web scraping is not a passive collection but an active one. As a result, informed consent is needed. Hogue also reported that many private companies have terms of use on their websites, which say no scraping, no crawling, no bots, etc. Government websites do not tend to have such restrictions. Since it would be burdensome to have researchers read all of the terms of use, Census is considering what they can do. She said that for now, Census is limiting the crawling and scraping to just federal state and local government websites.

Hogue said that the second policy issue is PII. She noted that the policy and legal people are very concerned about the unintentional scraping of PII. This raises questions about whether such a record would be a Title 13 record or a federal record. If it is, what are the disposal rules?

Hogue went on to describe the software product *Scraping Assisted by Learning* (SABLE), a collection of tools for crawling websites, scraping documents in data, and classifying the text. The models, which are based on text analysis and machine learning, are implemented using free, open-source Apache Nutch and Python.

SABLE has three main tasks: SABLE will crawl and scan the website, find the documents, and extract the text. Then a model is applied to determine whether the document is useful or not. If useful, it scrapes using a model to find the useful data and extract the numerical values and the corresponding text.

In order to move into a production environment, Census must have an authority to operate that requires a risk profile, a security assessment, documentation, audit trails, and subversion for code management. On August 22, 2019, SABLE was approved and ready for production. It is available on the Census Bureau's GitHub account.[4]

Census has used SABLE to seek out and collect information from state Comprehensive Annual Financial Reports (CAFR) and other online publications that contain tax revenue data. These CAFRs are used for much of the data that Census collects from state and local governments. Census used SABLE to crawl through state government sites, and found about 60,000 PDFs. Census staff manually evaluated a random sample of about 6,000 of them and manually put the sample through a useful/not-useful test. They then used this information to apply machine learning to build text classification models based on word sequences. There is no product based on this example, as yet.

Hogue said that they did the same thing on pension statistics data and are trying to release this as a product for the Bureau of Economic Analysis (BEA). BEA asked Census to scrape service costs and interest statistics found on the CAFRs. A two-stage approach of first finding the tables using word sequences and then applying a scraping algorithm was used to accomplish the task.

Hogue said that Census analysts also rely on Securities and Exchange Commission (SEC) filing data, online databases of financial reports for

[4] See https://www.github.com/uscensusbureau/SABLE programs, supplementary files, examples, and documentation.

publicly traded companies. Now analysts do not know when new reports are posted. Census has a Really Simple Syndication (RSS) feed that provides information on recent SEC filings. There is a current project to query this RSS feed to determine filing dates for various types of reports and to package it into a useful product for Census analysis.

Another scraping project is to target data in online building permit jurisdiction databases. Census releases construction indicators, such as housing starts, based on their Building Permits Survey (BPS), its Survey of Construction (SOC), and Nonresidential Coverage Evaluation (NCE). Information on new privately owned construction is often available in building permit databases. A few years ago, Census investigated the feasibility of using publicly available building permit data to supplement these surveys. It started in Chicago and Seattle, two cities with permit data available through APIs. The initial research showed that the data were very timely and of high quality. The problem was that there were many differences in the definitions used by different jurisdictions and not enough detail to actually use what would be scraped. It waited a few years and looked at seven more jurisdictions. The data are available in many different formats, but the classifications are becoming more standard. There is still a lack of information on housing units.

Hogue summarized by saying the challenges to using the building permits data are their representativeness and their inconsistency in terminology and formats. Census continues to explore the quality of scraped data by comparing them to survey data, and it is also looking at third-party data sources, such as Zillow and Construction Monitor.

Hogue said that the next step is to use SABLE in production, and to release a data product based in part on scraped data. Census would like to develop the SEC filing product, discussed above. After that, next steps will be guided by a new working group to address policy issues regarding web scraping and web crawling.

Hague briefly summarized the third party data that Census has used. It has looked at retailer data from NPD, both in aggregate and individual company data. NPD includes more than 1,300 retailers, both brick and mortar and e-commerce, and collects point-of-sale data. NPD captures some retailers that do not report to Census. The aggregate NPD data did not track well with Census estimates. However, the individual company data looked pretty good. Census is beginning to this examine data to impute for survey nonresponse.

Hogue went on to describe Census's use of credit card raw data. She said those data are perfect. The problem was that the company had a change in leadership and decided that it did not want to share its data with Census anymore.

The final third-party data she described is credit/debit/gift card process data. Census is trying to use the information to provide more geographic granularity for the monthly retail trade survey. It has purchased raw data, but there was a lot of suppression. It will be able to use the data in a product soon.

Hogue concluded by summarizing some of the issues and challenges with using third-party data: acquiring these data can take a long time, costs are not fixed—they can increase or decrease due to change in management or other company practices, the lack of transparent methods used to collect and clean these data, the quality of these data can be difficult to judge, and disclosure avoidance policies can be difficult to discern.

C.4. MEETING AGENDA

Panel on Improving USDA's Consumer Data for Food and Nutrition Policy Research
Third Meeting, September 21, 2018

The National Academy of Sciences Building, Room 120
2101 Constitution Ave NW, Washington, DC

Open Session

9:00 Plan for the day, goals for the meeting and of the panel more broadly
- **Marianne Bitler**, *Chair*

9:10 Update on recent developments at ERS and with FoodAPS-2
- **Jay Variyam, Mark Denbaly**, ERS

9:30 Improving data for policy research. For this session, researchers are asked to discuss their ideas for improving food and nutrition data—including integration of commercial and administrative data—to inform key policy issues.

- The value (and limits) of linking SNAP administrative data with other types of administrative data (unemployment Insurance, Medicaid, K-12 education) as well as the limits of existing survey data.
  - **Colleen Heflin**, Syracuse University
- Use of retail panel loyalty card data and Rhode Island state administrative records (housed in a secure facility at Brown University) to analyze how SNAP benefits are spent. Evidence needed to design a "smarter SNAP"
  - **Justine Hastings**, Brown University

- Understanding/assessing the quality of administrative SNAP data used in FoodAPS. Broader thoughts on food consumption data needs for obesity and other health research.
  - **Chuck Courtemanche**, Georgia State University
- Open discussion

11:15 Data Integration and linkages for policy research, use of administrative data

There is high value to ERS's Consumer Food Data System of linkages to external data sets—e.g., to NHANES, Nielsen datasets, IRI datasets, SNAP administrative data, CPS, SIPP, ACS, BRFSS, CEX, Nationwide Food Consumption Survey, PSID, state and local-level datasets with information on low-income households, etc. During this session, we discuss practices being developed by the statistical agencies for combining data sources.

- Administrative data linkages in the federal statistical system; the Next-Generation Data Platform—a collaboration between Census, ERS and FNS that links SNAP (19 States and 39 counties in CA) and WIC data (11 states) to Census survey data and administrative data: 17 State TANF agencies, VA, HUD and HHS data (Medicare and Medicaid) in a secure environment (described in the White paper provided to the panel).
  - **Amy O'Hara**, panel member and Georgetown University, will introduce the topic, highlighting strengths and weakness, potential and limitations, of statistical agency data linking approaches.
  - **Rachel Shattuck**, Census Bureau, to present views on the quality and utility of what ERS calls the Next-Generation Data Platform, challenges you see for the project going forward, and how the partners ERS/FNS and Census could improve it in the future.
  - **John Eltinge**, Census Bureau, to discuss interagency workshops and explorations related to quality issues associated with using multiple data sources (including proprietary data).
- Record Linkage programs at NCHS. NCHS has developed a record linkage program designed to maximize the scientific value of the Center's population-based surveys. Linked data files create new data resources that can support research to inform the development and evaluation of public health programs and policies. The focus of this presentation will be on existing linkages between NCHS national

population health surveys, such as the National Health Interview Survey (NHIS) and the National Health and Nutrition Examination Survey (NHANES), and administrative data collected from the Department of Housing and Urban Development's (HUD) largest housing assistance programs including, the Housing Choice Voucher program, federally supported public housing, and privately owned, subsidized multifamily housing. The presentation will include an assessment of the concordance between survey and administrative data sources and present results from studies looking at comparisons of health characteristics between persons receiving housing assistance and those who do not.

- **Cordell Golden** *(for Lisa Mirel)* NCHS

1:30 Additional non-government sources for filling data gaps in ERS's Consumer Food Data System program

- Feeding America—Collaborates with Urban Institute on a research program that attempts to detail the frequency of visits to food pantries by individuals, either as a temporary, emergency food source or as a regular supplemental food source. Feeding America also has a program to study the effectiveness and efficiency of a range of program interventions. What data do they use; what data do they produce; what are the unmet data needs.
  - **Rob Santos**, Urban Institute. Member of Feeding America Technical Advisory Group
- Improving geospatial information in ERS's food data system (for example, for assessing the role of accessibility of food outlets role in SNAP participation and effectiveness)
  - **Alessandro Bonanno**, Colorado State University
- Open discussion

2:30 Using proprietary data for food policy research

- Types, sources, and considerations in using store scanner data, household scanner data, and nutrition data from labels for food policy research. Presentation is based on researching statistical properties of the data; investigating sources, coverage, and uses of the data; and conducting analyses.
  - **Mary Muth**, RTI
- Understanding WIC issues with proprietary (scanner) data. Comments as a long time user of ERS Consumer Food

Data; ideas about how the data system should evolve over the next decade.
- **Helen Jensen,** Iowa State

- The Census Bureau's work on improving economic statistics through web scraping and machine learning to discover, collect, and process data from the web.
  - **Carma Hogue,** U.S. Census Bureau
- Open discussion

4:00 *Adjourn*

Appendix D

Biographical Sketches of Panel Members

MARIANNE P. BITLER (*Chair*) is a professor in the Department of Economics at the University of California, Davis. Dr. Bitler's expertise lies in public economics, labor economics, health economics, and applied microeconomics, with particular emphasis on the effects of government safety net programs on disadvantaged groups. Prior to arriving at UC Davis, she was a professor of economics at UC Irvine. She has worked at the Public Policy Institute of California, the RAND Corporation, the Board of Governors of the Federal Reserve System, and the Federal Trade Commission. Dr. Bitler is a research associate with the National Bureau of Economic Research and a research fellow at the Institute of Labor Economics (IZA) in Bonn, Germany. She has served on the National Academies' Health and Medicine Division Panel to Review the WIC Food Package and on the just completed Committee on National Statistics Panel to Review and Evaluate the 2014 Survey of Income and Program Participation's Content and Design. Dr. Bitler holds a Ph.D. from the Massachusetts Institute of Technology.

TIM BEATTY is a professor in the Department of Agricultural and Resource Economics at the University of California, Davis. Prior to joining UC Davis, he was a faculty member in the Department of Applied Economics at the University of Minnesota, and he has held visiting positions with the University of British Columbia, Statistics Norway, and the University of Bologna. His research relates to the empirical analysis of consumption behavior, in particular as it relates to health outcomes at both the household and aggregate levels. He has served as a co-editor of the *American Journal of Agricultural Economics*. He is a long-time member of the Agricultural and Applied Economics Association, serving in leadership roles in the Food Safety and Nutrition and Econometrics sections. He holds an M.Sc. in applied economics from the École des Hautes Études Commerciales de Montréal and a Ph.D. in agricultural and resource economics from the University of California, Berkeley.

F. **JAY BREIDT** is a professor in the Department of Statistics at Colorado State University, where he served from 2005 to 2010 as department chair. Dr. Breidt joined the Colorado State faculty in 2002 after nearly 10 years in the Department of Statistics at Iowa State University. His research interests include estimation for complex surveys, survey sampling, time series, and environmental monitoring. He is an associate editor of the *Electronic Journal of Statistics* and the *Journal of Forecasting*. He has previously served on several National Academies committees, including the Panel on Using ACS to Estimate Children in Poverty for School Breakfast and Lunch Programs and the Panel on the Census Bureau's Reengineered Survey of Income and Program Participation. Dr. Breidt is a fellow of the American Statistical Association and an elected member of the International Statistical Institute. He holds an M.S. and a Ph.D., both in statistics, from Colorado State University.

CRAIG GUNDERSEN is Soybean Industry Endowed Professor of Agricultural Strategy in the Department of Agricultural and Consumer Economics at the University of Illinois. Prior to joining the University of Illinois, he served as an economist at the U.S. Department of Agriculture's Economic Research Service as well as academic positions at Iowa State University. His research attempts to inform policy makers and program administrators who are seeking paths to reduce food insecurity and its consequences, with emphasis on food assistance programs, particularly the Supplemental Nutrition Assistance Program (SNAP). Dr. Gundersen serves as an editor for the *Journal of Nutrition* and the *American Journal of Agricultural Economics*. He holds a Ph.D. from the University of California, Riverside.

MICHAEL W. LINK is division vice president for Data Science, Surveys and Enabling Technologies at Abt Associates. Prior to joining Abt, he was chief methodologist for research methods at The Nielsen Company. He has a broad base of experience in survey research, having worked in academia (University of South Carolina), not-for-profit research (RTI International), government (Centers for Disease Control and Prevention), and the private sector (Nielsen). His research concerns some of the most pressing issues facing survey research, including techniques for improving survey participation and data quality, methodological issues involving use of multiple modes in data collection, and obtaining participation from hard-to-survey populations.

His research articles have appeared in *Public Opinion Quarterly* and other leading scientific journals. In 2011, he and several research colleagues received AAPOR's Warren J. Mitofsky Innovators Award for their work on address-based sampling designs. His current research focuses on emerging technologies, such as mobile and social platforms, as vehicles for measuring and understanding public attitudes and behaviors. He received his Ph.D. in political science from the University of South Carolina.

BRUCE D. MEYER is the McCormick Foundation professor of public policy in the Harris School of Public Policy Studies at the University of Chicago. Prior to this appointment he was a professor in the Economics Department at Northwestern University, where he taught for 17 years. His current research includes studies of poverty and inequality, government safety net programs, welfare policy, unemployment insurance, workers' compensation, disability, the health care safety net, labor supply, and the accuracy of household surveys. Previously, he was a visiting faculty member at Harvard University, University College London, and Princeton University. He is a research associate of the National Bureau of Economic Research and a member of the National Academy of Social Insurance and the Conference on Research on Income and Wealth. Dr. Meyer has served as an advisor to the U.S. Department of Labor, U.S. Bureau of Labor Statistics, New York State Office of Temporary and Disability Assistance, Human Resources Development Canada, Manpower Demonstration Research Corporation, and Mathematica Policy Research. He holds an M.A. from Northwestern University and a Ph.D. from the Massachusetts Institute of Technology, both in economics.

AMY B. O'HARA is a research professor in the Massive Data Institute and executive director of the Federal Statistical Research Data Center at the McCourt School for Public Policy at Georgetown University. She was previously a senior research scholar at the Stanford Institute for Economic Policy Research (2017–2018). From 2014 until her move to Stanford, she was chief of the Center for Administrative Records Research and Applications (CARRA), which was then part of the research and methodology directorate at the U.S. Census Bureau. She began her career at the Census Bureau in 2004 as an economist/statistician in the Social, Economic, and Housing Statistics Division before shifting to CARRA in 2008. Among other accomplishments in attempting to integrate administrative records data into the full suite of Census Bureau processes, she led the 2010 Census Match Study—an unprecedented complete match/linkage of the full set of returns from the 2010 decennial census to a composite of administrative records data from eight federal agencies. She received an Arthur S. Flemming Award for outstanding achievement and leadership in federal government service, from the Trachtenberg School of Public Policy and Public Administration, George Washington University, in 2012. She holds M.A. and Ph.D. degrees in economics, both from the University of Notre Dame.

ERIC B. RIMM is a professor of epidemiology and nutrition and director of the Program in Cardiovascular Epidemiology at the Harvard School of Public Health and a professor of medicine at the Harvard Medical School. His research group has specific interests both in the study of modifiable lifestyle choices (e.g., diet and physical activity) in relation to cardiovascular disease as well as the translation of these findings into public health interventions that are effective for schoolchildren, adults, and the food-insecure. He has previously served on the scientific advisory committee for the 2010 *U.S. Dietary Guidelines for Americans*. He has published more than 450 peer-reviewed publications during his 20-plus years on the faculty at Harvard. Dr. Rimm is an associate editor for the *American Journal of Clinical Nutrition* and the *American Journal of Epidemiology*. He also was awarded the 2012 American Society for Nutrition General Mills Institute of Health and Nutrition Innovation Award. He holds an Sc.D. in epidemiology from the Harvard School of Public Health.

NORA CATE SCHAEFFER is Sewell Bascom Professor of Sociology at the University of Wisconsin-Madison, where she also serves as faculty director of the University of Wisconsin Survey Center, teaches courses in survey research methods, and conducts research on questionnaire design and interaction during survey interviews. She currently serves as a member of the Public Opinion Quarterly Advisory Board of the American Association for Public Opinion Research and as a member of the General Social Survey Board of Overseers. She recently completed terms as the Council on Sections Representatives for the Survey Research Methods Section of the American Statistical Association and as a member of the Census Advisory Committee of Professional Associations. She is an elected fellow of the American Statistical Association. She has served on multiple National Academies committees, including seven consensus studies, and is a former member of the Committee on National Statistics. She holds a Ph.D. in sociology from the University of Chicago.

DIANE W. SCHANZENBACH is director of the Institute for Policy Research, the Margaret Walker Alexander Professor in the School of Education and Social Policy, and faculty fellow at Northwestern University. She is also currently research associate of the National Bureau of Economic Research, a senior fellow at The Brookings Institution, a visiting scholar at the Federal Reserve Bank of Chicago, and a faculty affiliate in the Institute for Research on Poverty at the University of Wisconsin. She studies policies aimed at improving the lives of children in poverty, including education, health, and income support policies. Her recent work has focused on tracing the impact of major public policies such as Supplemental Nutrition Assistance Program (SNAP) and early childhood education on children's long-term outcomes. She holds M.A. and Ph.D. degrees from Princeton University, both in economics.

SOFIA BERTO VILLAS-BOAS is a professor in the Department of Agricultural and Resource Economics at the University of California, Berkeley. Her research interests include industrial organization, consumer behavior, food policy, and environmental regulation. Her recent empirical work estimates the effects of policies on consumer behavior, such as a bottled water tax, a plastic bag ban, and a soda tax campaign and its implementation. Other published work has focused on the economics behind legislation banning wholesale price discrimination, contractual relationships along a vertical supply chain, including the role of those contracts in explaining pass-through of cost shocks along the supply chain into the retail prices that consumers face. She has been widely published in top economics and field journals, including the *Review of Economic Studies, Rand Journal of Economics, American Journal of Agricultural Economics, Journal of Environmental Economics and Management*, and *Marketing Science*. She holds a Ph.D. from the University of California, Berkeley in economics.

PARKE E. WILDE is professor at the Friedman School of Nutrition Science and Policy at Tufts University. His research focus is on U.S. food and nutrition policy, consumer economics, and federal food assistance programs. His current and past research has addressed the Supplemental Nutrition Assistance Program's Healthy Incentive Pilot; the geography of local food retail; federal commodity checkoff programs; and food and beverage marketing to children. He has also authored a textbook on food policy in the United States. Dr. Wilde was a member of the National Academies' Food Forum from 2011 to 2014 and served on the planning committee for a National Academies workshop on Sustainable Diets: Food for Healthy People and a Healthy Planet (2013). He holds a B.A. in political science from Swarthmore College and M.S. and Ph.D. degrees in agricultural economics from Cornell University.

JAMES P. ZILIAK is Carol Martin Gatton Endowed Chair in Microeconomics in the Department of Economics at the University of Kentucky and founding director of the Center for Poverty Research. His research expertise is in the areas of tax and welfare policy, poverty, and food insecurity. He is the principal investigator on the Research Program on Childhood Hunger funded by the U.S. Department of Agriculture's Food and Nutrition Service. He was a member of the National Academies' Health and Medicine Division Committee on the Examination of the Adequacy of Food Resources and SNAP Allotments, as well as its Committee on National Statistics Panel on the Review and Evaluation of the 2014 Survey of Income and Program Participation Content and Design. Dr. Ziliak has served as a visiting scholar at the Brookings Institution and as a visiting professor at University College London and the universities of Michigan and Wisconsin. He served as chair of the Committee on National Statistics' Workshop on an Agenda for Child Hunger and Food Insecurity Research. He holds M.A. and Ph.D. degrees in economics from India.

COMMITTEE ON NATIONAL STATISTICS

The Committee on National Statistics was established in 1972 at the National Academies of Sciences, Engineering, and Medicine to improve the statistical methods and information on which public policy decisions are based. The committee carries out studies, workshops, and other activities to foster better measures and fuller understanding of the economy, the environment, public health, crime, education, immigration, poverty, welfare, and other public policy issues. It also evaluates ongoing statistical programs and tracks the statistical policy and coordinating activities of the federal government, serving a unique role at the intersection of statistics and public policy. The committee's work is supported by a consortium of federal agencies through a National Science Foundation grant, a National Agricultural Statistics Service cooperative agreement, and several individual contracts.